"Those who think they have not time for bodily exercise will sooner or later have to find time for illness."

— Edward Stanley, the 15th Earl of Derby,
late 19th century

HOLD ON TO YOUR
MUSCLE
BE FREE OF DISEASE

Tom,

Merry Christmas &
Happy New Year

Cousin Bobby

HOLD ON TO YOUR
MUSCLE
BE FREE OF DISEASE

OPTIMIZE YOUR MUSCLE MASS TO BATTLE AGING AND DISEASE WHILE PROMOTING TOTAL FITNESS AND WEIGHT LOSS

ROBERT IAFELICE, MS, RDN

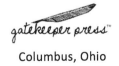
gatekeeper press™

Columbus, Ohio

Hold On to Your MUSCLE, Be Free of Disease: OPTIMIZE YOUR MUSCLE MASS TO BATTLE AGING AND DISEASE WHILE PROMOTING TOTAL FITNESS AND LASTING WEIGHT LOSS

Published by Gatekeeper Press
2167 Stringtown Rd, Suite 109
Columbus, OH 43123-2989
www.GatekeeperPress.com

The editorial work for this book are entirely the product of the author. Gatekeeper Press did not participate in and is not responsible for any aspect of this elements.

Library of Congress Control Number: 2022940165

Copyright for the images:

DM7/shutterstock.com
Vac1/shutterstock.com

ISBN (paperback): 9781662929229
eISBN: 97816w62929236

To the memory of my beloved father, Elio Iafelice, a good Christian man who, though beset by physical misfortune throughout his senior years, accepted and carried his cross, making the most of what God gave him...and to my dearest mother, Ameriga, whose selfless love and unending care for my father endured into her 90s.

Contents

PART III
How to Preserve and Strengthen Your Muscle Mass

Introduction

You might presume that a book about muscle would target athletes or anyone interested in bodybuilding or exercise performance. While it's true that athletes can certainly benefit from the latest scientific discoveries and simple lifestyle changes we'll be discussing, this book goes far beyond sports and bodybuilding or even just cosmetic appeal—this information is aimed at anyone who wants to achieve or maintain optimal health and evade the age-related degenerative diseases of our modern world.

Most of today's headlines about health and disease prevention are fixated on excess body weight and body fat and give little attention to muscle. For most people, muscle doesn't come to mind when discussing ways to help prevent the major killer diseases such as cancer, heart disease, diabetes, and Alzheimer's disease. Nor do people generally associate muscle with living longer.

So how *is* your muscle mass associated with preventing disease and extending your healthspan?

The answers you'll find in this book will transform your way of thinking about health and fitness. You'll understand that it's more about being *undermuscled* rather than just overly fat. You'll learn that muscle is a fundamental pillar of health and vitality. You'll discover the fascinating inherent mechanisms we've evolved to preserve this overlooked but extremely vital organ and how you can maximize the effectiveness of those mechanisms.

Our muscle mass is indispensable! It's not (necessarily) about building larger muscles—it's about the critical importance of preserving your muscle mass and strength as well as muscle quality throughout the course of your life. When your muscle mass or function is compromised or diminished, there's an obvious outcome in the form of *loss of functionality* and a not-so-obvious outcome in the form of *impaired metabolic health*. This dichotomy concerning the physiological effects of muscle—functionality and metabolic health—underscores the crucial role that muscle plays in health, fitness, and disease resistance. Furthermore, having more muscle mass as well as better muscle *quality* serves as a "metabolic reserve" that enables you to better withstand and recover from major stresses such as trauma and surgery and wasting diseases such as cancer. In fact, among older adults, greater muscle mass predicts longevity.[1]

Of course, when it comes to muscle health, exercise is king. The adage "Use it or lose it!" certainly applies here. Conventional wisdom says that over time, we should progressively lose functionality and suffer from the expected aches and pains associated with advancing age. But age-related functional impairment is not inevitable! We have the genetic potential to sustain complete functionality throughout our lives. ***We don't slow down because we're getting old—we get old because we slow down.***[2]

After reading this book, you'll gain a greater appreciation for resistance exercise and understand why it should be a mainstay of everyone's fitness program. You'll learn that brief stints of high-intensity exercise provide more substantial benefits than continuous, steady-state exercise does. I'll clear up the confusion about protein and reveal the truth about how much, how often, and what types of protein are best for muscle optimization.

All that said, it's not just about exercise and protein! Remarkably, simply eating less often and/or minimizing your carbohydrate intake can actually mimic *some* of the effects of exercise and exert a powerful effect on muscle tissue maintenance. This book will also teach you how to weed out the hype from the truly effective dietary supplements such as creatine that have been proven to benefit muscle mass and function.

Ultimately, all roads lead to muscle, which is why it's not surprising that most of today's popular lifestyle interventions intersect with our muscle. A multifactorial approach integrating the *right* exercise, the *right* diet, and the *right* supplements will lay out the ideal path toward having optimal muscle mass and therefore overall health enhancement.

I've packed this book with valuable information to help people of all ages improve their health and maintain those improvements. The earlier you incorporate these recommendations, the better you'll feel today and in the long term. Nevertheless, aging adults will benefit the most from this book because they are battling a new nemesis: sarcopenia. Sarcopenia is the gradual loss of muscle mass and strength with age.

After age 30, you begin to lose as much as 3% – 5% of muscle mass per decade. Unfortunately, just at a time in your life when you have a more pressing need to shore up your muscle health, your normal exercise and dietary routines become less effective precisely as a consequence of your advancing age. Similar to a football team losing at halftime, aging adults need to make "adjustments" during the second half of life in order to turn the tide in their favor. This book will teach you how to make those all-important exercise and dietary adjustments to push back on muscle loss and functional aging.

So let's begin a journey to discover why muscle is the key organ in our bodies that drives robust health and healthy aging—and how we can all build, protect, and sustain it.

PART I

Why is Muscle so Critically Important for Our Health?

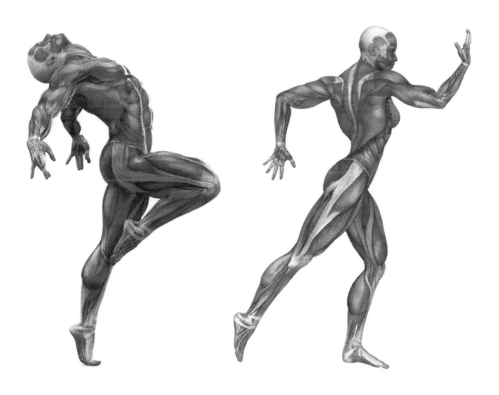

Chapter 1

Functionality – The Obvious

The primary focus of this book is the more than 600 skeletal muscles in our bodies.[3] Connected to our bones by tendons, skeletal muscles (referred to henceforth as just "muscle") are the muscles that we control. They are essential for physical performance—they work in tandem with our bones to enable us to stand, walk, run, ride a bicycle, dance, lift things, swim, chew, swallow, etc. Muscle is often likened to a mechanical engine, and a very efficient and powerful one at that. When corrected for weight differences, the power output of an automobile engine is only 1½ times greater than that of a muscle.[4]

Sarcopenia

While we take our ability to perform daily activities for granted, we also assume that our functional capacity will gradually deteriorate as we age. (But it doesn't have to! See Part III.) Sarcopenia—the age-related loss of muscle *mass* and muscle *strength*—is a major determinant of impaired functionality in older adults. There is also a progressive decline in the *quality* of muscle with advancing age.[5] Muscle quality explains why larger muscles (i.e., muscles of greater mass) are not necessarily stronger. Indeed, smaller muscles with better muscle quality have the ability to generate more force and are thus stronger. However, several factors including infiltration of fat within muscle fibers can lessen the quality of muscle (see Chapter 7 for more on muscle quality).[6]

Sarcopenia predominantly affects older adults. However, similar to dementia and osteoporosis, sarcopenia has been observed in younger adults as well.[7] Beginning as early as age 30 (if someone is not active), sarcopenia progresses gradually, until it accelerates after the fifth decade of life. In fact, in severe instances, 30% – 40% of muscle can be lost between the ages of 50 and 80.[8] This is especially disturbing when you consider that muscle makes up about 40% of total body mass![9]

Sarcopenia is a significant public health issue worldwide. It has a prevalence of 5% – 13% among people aged 60 – 70 years and up to 50% in people over 80 years of age. Although it already afflicts more than 50 million people today, sarcopenia is projected to afflict more than 200 million people in the next 40 years.[5]

While for some people sarcopenia is confined to moderately diminished physical competency, in others, it can lead to a reduced quality of life, a loss of independence, a need for long-term care, and physical disability.[10] Simply getting out of a chair or walking up steps may become challenging when muscle mass and strength are diminished. Frailty—characterized by increased vulnerability to minor stressors—is common among people with sarcopenia.[5]

Frailty is especially common in people who have both sarcopenia and osteoporosis. Bone is strengthened when voluntary forces (or mechanical loading) are applied on the bone. Bone cells (mainly osteocytes) sense those high forces and respond by increasing bone formation and bone density.[11] *The maximum forces acting on bone are created by muscle. Since people with sarcopenia have low muscle mass and strength, they will tend to also have weaker bones.* Thus, sarcopenia and osteoporosis are comorbid disorders, which is to say that they often coexist.[8] The term "osteosarcopenia" has been coined to describe this condition, which is characterized by the infiltration of fat into both muscle and bone.[12] Interestingly, both of these conditions are linked to inadequate dietary protein (see Chapter 8). Unlike osteoporosis, however, public health campaigns to raise awareness of sarcopenia are lacking.[13]

Sarcopenia often coexists with osteoarthritis as well.[14] With less muscle to cushion force and impact, joint pain is intensified. Over time, the wear and tear of the joints and ligaments may become crippling. This leads to a vicious cycle of less exercising and further muscle (and bone) loss. All in all, it is evident that muscle, bone, and joints are considerably intertwined.

The complex burden of sarcopenia on public health

Reprinted with permission from Beaudart et al.: Sarcopenia: burden and challenges for public health. Archives of Public Health 2014 72:45.

Metabolic Reserve

As a stockpile of protein for energy production, muscle plays a critical role during illness. When energy demands are high (e.g., infections, multiple traumas, burns, fever) or when energy is depleted (e.g., general loss of appetite, cancer cachexia or "wasting"), amino acids that result from the breakdown of muscle protein are burned for energy.[15] Low muscle quality and quantity are associated with higher death rates in intensive care unit (ICU) patients. Functional impairment that persists after critical illness as well as after a variety of surgical complications is also linked to having low muscle mass.[16] In other words, greater muscle mass can be a lifesaver!

As part of an assessment to determine patients' metabolic reserve and "fitness" prior to surgery and during recovery from ICU care, innovative techniques are currently being utilized and investigated that would identify patients with low muscle quality and quantity. Glycogen—the storage form of carbohydrates—is a vital energy source (though a limited one) for critically ill patients, and its content in muscle may also reflect a patient's metabolic reserve. Depletion of muscle glycogen stores results in severe muscle damage. Why? Because rather than glycogen being broken down for energy, muscle protein must be broken down.

In ICU patients, muscle glycogen reaches the brink of complete exhaustion within just hours of the patient having been admitted. This leads to poor muscle recovery and regeneration, resulting in devastating outcomes. For the sake of comparison, muscle glycogen stores in elite endurance athletes (e.g., prolonged bike racing competitors) are far from being completely depleted (see graph below). Thus, in terms of glycogen depletion, being in the ICU may be likened to running multiple marathons.[16,17]

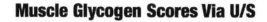

Muscle Glycogen Scores Via U/S

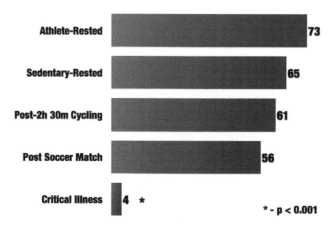

Muscle glycogen scores via ultrasound (U/S)

Reprinted with permission from: Wischmeyer P.E., San-Millan I. Winning the war against ICU-acquired weakness: New innovations in nutrition and exercise physiology. Crit. Care. 2015;19(Suppl. 3):S6.

Patients at high risk of malnutrition in particular may benefit from pre-surgery or pre-illness nutrition and exercise interventions.[17] We'll discuss those in ensuing chapters. Such interventions feature intense resistance exercise and the consumption of high-quality animal protein, both of which can drive muscle gains when repeated over time and in tandem. The payoff is a larger reserve of muscle (as well as muscle glycogen) that will support the metabolic demands of a patient who is critically ill.

Assessment of muscle health and function is also recommended as a preventive strategy in healthy adults. A position paper published in 2019 by experts from the WHO and other medical organizations encourages clinicians and general practitioners to routinely assess older adults for declines in muscle strength and physical performance that predict future falls, fractures, and care dependence.[18] The most widely applicable tests recommended by the experts for use in daily clinical practice are the handgrip test for muscle strength and gait speed for physical performance. These assessments of muscle strength and performance would be a fitting complement to the American Heart Association's recommendation of routinely evaluating cardiorespiratory fitness in primary care (see Chapter 2).

At this point, we've taken a very brief look at the more familiar functions of our undervalued muscle. In Chapter 2, we'll dive into a more elaborate discussion of the extraordinary but lesser-known role of muscle in regulating whole-body metabolic health and longevity. Part II will describe the causes of muscle loss, while Part III will present effective muscle-preserving strategies that you can immediately and easily integrate into your lifestyle.

Chapter 2

Metabolic Health – The Less Obvious

Metabolic diseases are characterized by the abnormal metabolism of proteins, fats, and/or carbohydrates. They also feature impaired functioning of mitochondria, the power plants in our cells that convert fuel and oxygen into most of the cell's energy. The chronic conditions that fall into the rubric of metabolic disorder traditionally include diabetes, obesity, cardiovascular diseases, and cancer.[1] With Alzheimer's disease now being regarded as a metabolic disorder as well,[2] all of today's top killer diseases are thus accounted for. Collectively, the sharp rise in the incidence of these metabolic disorders undermines the present and future health and well-being of the global population.[3] Data from the 2009 – 2016 National Health and Nutrition Examination Survey (NHANES) indicate that the number of American adults who are metabolically *healthy* (including those who are not overweight) is strikingly low and constitutes a serious public health concern.[4]

Muscle plays a central though underappreciated role in metabolic health and the prevention of metabolic diseases. But before we examine the muscle-disease connection, let's first take a quick look at the broader context of physical fitness. Changes in muscle mass affect body composition, and body composition is one of the five components of cardiorespiratory (aerobic) fitness. Does just being physically fit affect your risk of disease?

Cardiorespiratory Fitness (CRF) and Risk of Disease

Worldwide, about 1 of every 3 adults is physically *inactive*. That means that they do not meet the World Health Organization (WHO) recommendations of a minimum of 150 minutes per week of moderate to vigorous aerobic physical activity.[5] Among these people who do not exercise regularly, a perception persists that as long as a person avoids the traditional risk factors (e.g., smoking, obesity, high cholesterol) and passes a yearly physical, there's no need to exercise. Provided they aren't overweight, these individuals presume there's no urgency to work out and improve their cardiorespiratory fitness (CRF). "My doctor says my heart is strong, so why subject myself to the misery of exercise?" people might say. "After all, isn't being physically fit only necessary for competitive athletes? What does exercise have to do with cancer or Alzheimer's disease or diabetes?"

The short answer: *A lot!*

The importance of cardiorespiratory fitness extends far beyond its usefulness as a measurement of physical activity. Cardiorespiratory fitness is a powerful indicator of overall health! Though often overlooked, CRF may be the most important risk factor for cardiovascular diseases. Abundant evidence indicates that CRF is a major risk factor for dying from cardiovascular diseases and from *all* causes. CRF is strongly linked to mortality rates related to depression, dementia, and certain cancers, particularly those of the breast and colon/digestive tract.[6]

Remarkably, according to a policy statement from the American Heart Association, the ability of cardiovascular fitness to predict chronic disease and premature death is significantly more powerful than classical risk factors such as smoking, high blood pressure, elevated cholesterol, type 2 diabetes, and obesity![6]

Studies have consistently shown that both sedentary time (prolonged sitting) and poor CRF are potent and independent predictors of poor health and premature death.[7] A review of 47 studies found that even among people who exercise regularly, sedentary behavior was associated with an increased risk of death from cardiovascular disease, cancer, diabetes, and any cause. Notably, these adverse health effects were less pronounced in individuals who exercised more.[8] Breaking up sedentary time or replacing it with exercise and non-exercise activities (e.g., household chores, lawn and garden work, daily walking) improves cardiovascular health.[9]

Although cardiorespiratory fitness is invaluable to good health and longevity, it's the only major risk factor *not* included in routine clinical examinations in primary care. Strong evidence suggests that aerobic exercise testing should be conducted as a primary prevention assessment in much the same way that doctors test blood pressure, blood sugar, and cholesterol levels. In fact, the American Heart Association has released a statement recommending that an assessment of CRF be added to the vital signs obtained in standard clinical practice.[10]

Cardiorespiratory fitness is typically measured by VO2max, or maximal oxygen uptake. VO2max reflects the maximum capacity of the body to transport (via the circulation) and utilize oxygen during intense or maximal exercise. Regular exercise increases maximum oxygen consumption and thus improves physical fitness. VO2max can be measured either directly with an exercise test that requires maximal effort or indirectly during submaximal exercise testing. While the direct measurement of VO2max is clearly the most accurate method, it calls for specialized equipment and is usually restricted to clinical or research settings. Moreover, it carries a greater risk of adverse events in people with a history of cardiovascular disease. Submaximal exercise testing, on the other hand, is a more practical alternative to assess fitness in health/

fitness settings. It provides a reasonably accurate estimate of VO2max from the heart rate response to exercise that is less than maximal. Various modes of submaximal testing include using treadmills, stationary bicycles, and a simple step test.[11]

The Muscle-Disease Connection

Muscle contributes to the maintenance of optimal health in several different ways. The metabolic functions of muscle can be grouped into the following primary intersecting mechanisms of action:[12]

- Calorie burning
- Blood sugar control
- Metabolic flexibility
- Excretion of myokines

Calorie Burning

Muscle is a major determinant of the resting metabolic rate (RMR), which is the rate at which the body burns energy (calories) at complete rest. Muscle accounts for 20% – 30% of the RMR,[12] and the RMR is responsible for 60% – 80% of the total amount of calories you burn each day.[13] Having more muscle, then, enables your "metabolic engine" to keep firing and burn calories at a higher rate even when you're idle.

During exercise and other physical activities, muscle is harnessed to rev up calorie burning severalfold. Muscle's contribution to increasing energy expenditure is central to weight management and battling obesity. Obesity is described by the WHO as one of the most important emerging chronic diseases of the 21st century, in part because obesity raises the risk of other metabolic diseases such as type 2 diabetes and cardiovascular disease, thus shortening lifespans.[14]

Blood Sugar Control

The most common metabolic disorder is diabetes. Alarmingly, according to data collected from the National Health and Nutrition Examination Survey (NHANES), *more than half* of American adults in 2011 – 2012 had either diabetes or prediabetes![15] What's more, diabetes is a global epidemic. Currently, close to *half a billion* people on the planet are living with diabetes (type 1 and type 2 combined, although the vast majority of these cases are type 2, also called T2D).[16] Compared to adults without diabetes, adults with diabetes have a 50% higher risk of dying from any cause, not to mention the risk of multiple complications (e.g., visual impairment, renal failure, and leg amputation).[17] People with diabetes also have a reduced life expectancy of 4 – 8 years.[18]

[Note: This discussion is focused primarily on type 2 diabetes, the predominant form of diabetes (about 91% of adults) and the one that is lifestyle-related; type 1 diabetes is a much less prevalent autoimmune disorder.]

Elevated blood sugar and insulin resistance—we'll discuss the latter in coming chapters—are the hallmarks of diabetes. *As you will discover throughout this book, the ability of muscle to control blood sugar may be the most important role that muscle plays in supporting optimal metabolic health*. In order to fully appreciate the role that muscle plays in controlling blood sugar, you must first understand how extremely damaging excess blood sugar is to your health.

While maintaining healthy blood sugar levels will help keep diabetes at bay, it may also be the most effective dietary strategy we can use to prevent most of the other major metabolic diseases that threaten us. That's because faulty blood sugar metabolism may underlie many diseases. Chronically elevated blood sugar levels damage blood vessels and nerves throughout the body. For people with diabetes as well as prediabetes, the consequences are an increased risk of serious complications, including heart disease and stroke, blindness, kidney failure, neuropathy, infections, and nonalcoholic fatty liver disease.[19]

The association between type 2 diabetes and cardiovascular disease is especially profound. Compared to people without type 2 diabetes, a person with T2D has an approximate twofold increased risk of developing cardiovascular disease. That's the same risk as someone who's already had a previous heart attack.[20] Diabetes is also linked to many cancers and to a higher risk of dementia, particularly Alzheimer's disease. Alzheimer's disease is so closely linked to diabetes that it has been referred to as "type 3 diabetes."[21]

In 2019, half of the people with diabetes were undiagnosed.[22] These people can live without symptoms for many years—even decades—while excess blood glucose (sugar) is silently causing tremendous damage to their cells and tissues. Some individuals may develop symptoms but remain unaware that diabetes is the cause.

As we age, our ability to properly metabolize glucose progressively deteriorates and our blood levels of glucose (and insulin) become elevated. Compared to younger age groups, adults aged 60 and over are more than twice as likely to have diabetes (and this figure will continue to rise as the population ages).[23] The good news is that faulty glucose regulation is *not* an unavoidable consequence of aging. As you will soon see, muscle plays an essential role in preventing this.

Diabetes aside, everyone should always strive to maintain healthy blood sugar levels—this is perhaps the best predictor of a long life! Since we spend more than two-thirds of our day in a fed (nonfasting) state, spikes in blood sugar that occur *after* meals present a significant danger. Emerging evidence suggests that despite being short-lived, blood sugar spikes leave a long-lasting "imprint" in blood vessel cells that leaves a "legacy" for the future development of inflammation and disease even if/when good control of blood sugar is eventually achieved. This phenomenon is known as "metabolic memory" or the "legacy effect," and it suggests that early aggressive treatment of hyperglycemia (high blood sugar) is mandatory.[24] In short, keeping your blood sugar levels in a healthy range early on may prevent the sustained activation of pro-inflammatory genes triggered by hyperglycemia.

Our bodies tightly maintain and regulate normal levels of blood glucose because chronically elevated blood glucose is highly toxic to cells and tissues. One of the major mechanisms by which glucose wields its toxic effects in the body (glucotoxicity) is through a process called "glycation" and the associated formation of harmful molecules called "AGEs."

The AGEs That Age You

Glycation is an unwanted, uncontrolled reaction that occurs in the body between sugars and either proteins, fats, or DNA. When sugar sticks to these molecules, harmful compounds called "advanced glycation endproducts" or AGEs are formed in nearly every tissue and organ of the body. This process was originally identified over a century ago as a chemical rection known as the "Maillard reaction" that occurs in cooked foods. When specific proteins bond with sugars during high-temperature cooking (as well as food processing and storage), the same AGEs that form in our bodies are also responsible for the development of browning (caramelization) and the characteristic aromas of roasted, broiled, fried, baked, and grilled foods. Likewise, glycation in the body leads to a "caramelization" of our cells and tissues!

One of the ways that these AGEs wreak havoc in the body is by inducing crosslinks (a type of chemical bond) between molecules of long-lived proteins such as collagen, elastin, and lens proteins. Crosslinking causes the proteins to gum up and become structurally distorted, resulting in altered functioning. This cell-damaging process leads to increased stiffness and loss of elasticity in a variety of tissues. AGE-induced crosslinks manifest as wrinkling of skin, hardening of arteries, stiffening of joints, and clouding of the lens of the eye (cataracts). When DNA is targeted by glycation, mutations and potentially cancer may be the fallout. *AGEs can even damage muscle tissue and contribute to the loss of muscle mass and function as we age.*[21]

Ultimately, AGEs speed up aging—no acronym could be more appropriate! AGEs have been associated with aging and age-related diseases, including neurodegenerative disorders, atherosclerosis, renal failure, immunological changes, skin photoaging, osteoporosis, frailty, and increased risk of cancer and tumor progression. Not surprisingly, the aging effects of glycation are fast-tracked in diabetes.[21]

People with diabetes are especially vulnerable to the deleterious effects of glycation and AGEs. When blood sugar is chronically elevated (as it is in people with diabetes), the body's proteins have more time to come into contact with sugar molecules. Consequently, glycation is accelerated and more AGEs accumulate in tissues, contributing to diabetic complications such as retinopathy, neuropathy, kidney disease, and cardiovascular diseases. Glycation also impairs the signaling action of insulin, the hormone that lowers blood sugar. Insulin receptors on the surface of cell membranes are proteins that can be damaged by glycation, resulting in insulin not being able to bind as well to its receptors to initiate its signaling actions. (Think of these receptors as being docking stations.) Additionally, insulin itself is a protein whose structure can be warped through glycation. AGEs also exert toxic effects on the insulin-secreting beta cells of the pancreas.[21] Furthermore, a transport protein called GLUT4 that facilitates the diffusion of glucose into the cell may also be reduced in number by AGEs.[25] All of these effects of glycation undermine the ability of insulin to control blood sugar levels, thus contributing to hyperglycemia. Hyperglycemia in turn leads to more glycation and AGEs, creating a vicious cycle.

SUGAR + PROTEIN = AGEs

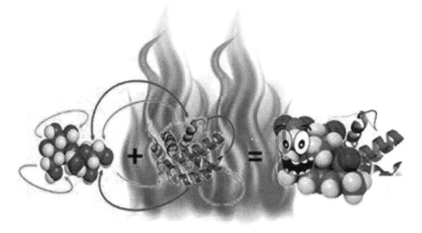

Image reproduced from original with permission from David P. Turner, Ph.D., Turner Research Lab, MUSC College of Medicine

As evidence of the harmful effects of glycation, the body is naturally equipped with defense mechanisms that detoxify and remove AGEs. Various enzyme systems in the body act to scavenge compounds that are direct precursors of AGEs (formed via sugar-protein glycation), thus preventing AGE formation. In fact, in diabetes, the production of these detoxifying enzymes is ramped up to counter the buildup of AGEs caused by chronically high blood sugar levels. Once AGEs are formed, they can also be broken down by protein-digesting enzymes called "proteases." Unfortunately, the capacity of this intrinsic defense system can be overwhelmed by increased formation of AGE precursor molecules (e.g., from excessive dietary carbohydrates), which then results in greater production of AGEs.[25]

Thus far, we've talked about glycation primarily in terms of its occurrence in the body when sugar molecules attach to proteins, fats, or DNA. That's because endogenous (inside the body) glycation and AGE formation are relevant to the role that muscle plays in regulating blood sugar. Nevertheless, it's important to note that exogenous (outside the body) formation of AGEs through the cooking and processing of food also contributes to serum levels of AGEs. (Interestingly, while fewer AGEs are found in low-fat vegan diets, the amount of AGEs in the plasma of vegans is higher than that of omnivores.[26]) There is an ongoing debate, however, as to whether dietary (exogenous) AGEs are retained in the body long enough to pose a risk to our health. More research is needed as current studies are controversial and conflicting.[27]

The Destructive Duo: Oxidative Stress and Inflammation

Not to be outdone by the AGE-ing of your body's tissues, excessive blood glucose (hyperglycemia) also leads to two nasty repercussions: oxidative stress and inflammation. While acute (short-term) inflammation is essential to the healing and repairing of injured or infected tissues, chronic low-grade inflammation that persists unresolved (a.k.a. "smolder") is not so good. Rather, it's pretty vicious. Prolonged, uncontrolled inflammation underlies the development of a wide variety of diseases, including neuro-degenerative disorders, cardiovascular diseases, diabetes, cancer, arthritis, osteoporosis, frailty, *sarcopenia,* and accelerated aging.[28]

The release of pro-inflammatory compounds (cytokines) that's prompted by hyperglycemia exerts systemic effects that ravage the entire body. High production of pro-inflammatory cytokines can cause DNA damage (mutations) and tissue destruction that may lead to irreversible organ malfunction. Inflammation caused by high blood sugar can then worsen blood sugar control by damaging the insulin-producing beta cells of the pancreas.[29] In another endless loop—one that very much fits in with the main focus of this book—high blood sugar resulting from muscle loss can ignite chronic inflammation...which subsequently leads to a further decline in muscle mass and strength.[30] More about that in a minute.

High blood glucose also causes increased production of reactive oxygen species (ROS). ROS are highly unstable molecules called "free radicals" that are primarily produced in the body as spinoffs of the chemical reactions in the cellular mitochondria that convert food and oxygen to energy. These free radicals are also known as "oxidants" because they trigger oxidation reactions similar to an apple browning or a nail rusting. (According to one theory of aging, our cells oxidize or "rust" over a lifetime due to the fact that we breathe in oxygen. In other words, what gives us life eventually causes our demise.[31]) At low levels, these biological free radicals provide health benefits such as defending against infectious agents. Indeed, free radicals induced by exercise play a role in mediating many of the beneficial adaptations we get from exercising. However, excessive concentrations of free radicals in the body can damage proteins, fats, and DNA.[32]

Fortunately, we're equipped with defense systems that can prevent or destroy excess free radicals. These defenses include endogenous antioxidants such as coenzyme Q10 (CoQ10) and glutathione as well as an arsenal of potent antioxidant enzymes. Among the many exogenous antioxidants we obtain from our food are vitamin C, vitamin E, carotenoids, flavonoids, zinc, and selenium. However, when excess production of ROS overwhelms antioxidant defenses, oxidative stress (cell and tissue damage) results.[33] Hyperglycemia not only increases the production of ROS, it also suppresses the antioxidant defense system, thus tilting the balance in favor of the development of oxidative stress.[32]

The degree of tissue damage caused by oxidative stress directly correlates with how long an individual's high blood glucose levels persist. That said, even daily acute fluctuations in blood glucose levels activate oxidative stress. Abundant evidence indicates that oxidative stress is involved in the onset and/or progression of major metabolic diseases such as cancer, cardiovascular diseases, and diabetes. It is particularly associated with diabetic complications and insulin resistance (see "Metabolic Flexibility").[32]

Like two sides of the same coin, chronic inflammation and oxidative stress are inextricably linked, occurring simultaneously in many chronic diseases. When inflammation is the primary disorder, oxidative stress develops as a secondary disorder and vice versa. In both instances, the two processes feed off each other to create a more damaging synergistic effect. In acute inflammation (e.g., injury or infection), ROS are liberated from immune cells partly to kill invading pathogens and resolve the inflammation. This is a short-lived event that is somewhat regulated by an increased production of antioxidants. In contrast, high blood glucose levels trigger the release of pro-inflammatory cytokines that generate a *continuous overproduction* of ROS. Paired with the depletion of antioxidants (also caused by hyperglycemia), this exaggerated production of ROS induces oxidative stress. By causing tissue injury, oxidative stress then induces the recruitment of inflammatory cells (to heal and repair) and cytokines. Both promote further inflammation, and a vicious cycle ensues. On top of that, all three mediators of glucotoxicity—oxidative stress, inflammation, and AGEs—interact with each other and spur each other on, causing a broader cycle of cellular damage.[32,34]

How Muscle Controls Blood Sugar: The Glucose Sink

You now have an appreciation of the considerable damage that excess blood sugar can elicit in the body. But the burning question remains: how exactly does muscle regulate blood glucose?

Since excessive glucose is so toxic, the body must have a place to dispose of the glut of glucose in the bloodstream. Following a meal, muscle is the primary "glucose sink" that takes up and stores the surplus glucose (up to 80% – 90%) in the blood and effectively uses it for energy, thus lowering blood glucose. For the most part, this uptake of surplus glucose into muscle is facilitated by the signaling action of the hormone insulin. When insulin binds to the insulin receptors on the surface of muscle cells, that action induces the glucose transporter GLUT4 to move from a storage site within the cell to the cell surface, where it enables glucose to enter the cell.[35] The more sensitive that muscle tissue is to insulin, the more effectively it uses insulin to clear excess glucose from the bloodstream. Also, increased insulin sensitivity means that less insulin is needed to generate its signaling effects. This is vitally important! Excessive insulin in the bloodstream (hyperinsulinemia) is linked to obesity and chronic diseases (see "Whey Protein" for more on the dangers of high insulin levels).

Increasing muscle mass above even average levels has been shown to boost insulin sensitivity and glucose uptake from the blood. More muscle bulk means more space is available for glucose to get into the cell, thereby heightening the insulin sensitivity (more insulin receptors) and insulin signaling that are needed to drive this process. This results in stable management of blood glucose levels. In fact, muscle enhancement has been associated with a striking 63% reduction in the prevalence of diabetes![36] Conversely, a *decrease* in muscle mass is a key factor in insulin *resistance*, which is the driving force behind type 2 diabetes and metabolic syndrome (see "Metabolic Flexibility"). Exercise—both aerobic exercise and resistance training—results in long-standing improvements in muscle insulin sensitivity and glucose regulation.[37]

Metabolic Flexibility

It's probably safe to say that most of us haven't given much thought to the fact that our bodies utilize different metabolic fuels for energy at different times. For example, we burn fat to fuel our muscles at rest or when walking slowly; however, we increasingly burn glucose (glycogen stores) as the intensity of physical activity increases. Metabolic flexibility is a relatively new term that describes the ability to periodically transition freely between our two primary fuels—glucose and fat—depending on supply and demand. From an evolutionary perspective, metabolic flexibility allowed early humans to withstand extreme fluctuations in fuel supply—they could store energy in the form of fat during times of food abundance and also function optimally during brief or prolonged periods of food scarcity.[38]

As both a major user and producer of the body's energy, muscle plays a key role in whole-body metabolic flexibility. A core characteristic of muscle is its ability to select fat or glucose as its main fuel. This intrinsic feature of muscle can be clearly demonstrated by comparing the metabolic flexibility of muscle in fit, lean individuals with that of sedentary, obese individuals. In people who are fit and lean, muscle efficiently burns glucose after eating but burns fat for fuel while fasting. This *appropriate* response to supply and demand keeps blood sugar under control after meals while also helping avoid sugar cravings when fasting (via breaking down stored fat for energy). In contrast, in people who are sedentary and obese, muscle is less able to clear away glucose in the blood after eating and has a diminished ability to burn stored fat while fasting.[39] This leads to poor blood sugar control characterized by frequent spikes and ensuing crashes, a roller coaster that results in constant hunger and a dependence on sugar- and carbohydrate-rich snacks to sustain energy levels.

The compromised metabolic flexibility (or metabolic *inflexibility*) of muscle in sedentary, obese individuals contributes to the accumulation of triglycerides (fat) within muscle cells, and that in turn interferes with insulin signaling and initiates or worsens insulin resistance.[40]

When muscle is resistant to insulin, the ability of insulin to facilitate the transfer of glucose from the bloodstream into muscle cells is impaired. Why? Because muscle cells are unable to "hear" the insulin signal and are thus unaffected by insulin's action. As a consequence of muscle's resistance to insulin, glucose cannot readily enter muscle cells. Blood glucose levels then rise. To counteract the reduced effectiveness of insulin in this scenario, the pancreas goes into overdrive and secretes increasingly more insulin in an effort to shove glucose into muscle cells and keep blood glucose levels in the normal range. These high blood levels of insulin—referred to as "hyperinsulinemia"—exacerbate insulin resistance because the muscle cells stop responding to the flood of insulin. Another vicious circle ensues, and this one drives the development or progression of metabolic diseases, primarily type 2 diabetes and metabolic syndrome.[41]

In a practical sense, insulin resistance is the same as carbohydrate intolerance. People who have insulin resistance tend to generate excessively elevated glucose and insulin levels in response to eating carbohydrates. On the other hand, in people who do not have insulin resistance, the glucose and insulin response to consuming carbohydrates is blunted. Basically, when your muscle cells are resistant to insulin, their ability to burn carbohydrates for energy is diminished in favor of efficiently converting carbohydrates to fat. This leads to the development of risk factors associated with insulin resistance syndrome, better known as "metabolic syndrome." These risk factors are abdominal obesity, hypertension, low levels of protective HDL, and elevated blood levels of triglycerides, glucose, and insulin.[42] Loss of muscle mass increases the risk of insulin resistance. However, as we've already noted, more muscle *increases* sensitivity to insulin and thus *reverses* insulin resistance.

Metabolic inflexibility and insulin resistance in muscle tissue are closely related defects in metabolism that are *acquired* defects. They are the consequences of our modern lifestyle, one that's marked primarily by inactivity and an abundance of convenient, quick-to-digest, high-sugar and high-calorie foods. These two distinct defects negatively impact **blood sugar control**, which of course is the focal point of the beneficial effects that muscle has on metabolic health.

Metabolic inflexibility and insulin resistance underlie many metabolic diseases, including metabolic syndrome, prediabetes, type 2 diabetes, cardiovascular diseases, and cancer. Disorders involving insulin resistance affect more than 100 million people in the United States.[42,43] More than 2 in 3 American adults are obese or overweight,[44] and they tend to be insulin-resistant. Moreover, insulin resistance is also observed in many people who don't have any major metabolic disorder (e.g., sedentary individuals), and it occurs in varying dgrees.[45,46] *In other words, all things considered, approximately 3 in 4 American adults are unable to efficiently process carbohydrates*[47] *and experience poor blood sugar control as the outcome.* These people may need to curb their daily carb consumption to 100 grams or even 40 grams (people's average daily carb consumption is 250 – 400 grams). Because individuals vary greatly as to what their suitable carb intake would be, pinning down the ideal carbohydrate consumption for a specific person is a matter of trial and error.

At the cellular level, data from recent studies strongly implicate *reduced muscle mitochondrial function* in the development of both metabolic inflexibility and insulin resistance. It appears that a heritable defect in the ability to oxidize (burn) fat in the mitochondria of muscle cells may initially trigger the development of inflexible muscle.[48] This may explain why metabolically inflexible individuals have difficulty burning fat during fasting or while eating diets low in calories/carbohydrates or high in fats. The reduced fat-burning capacity of muscle mitochondria results in the buildup of fat within the muscle, and that buildup drives the subsequent development of insulin resistance.[49]

So how do you restore metabolic flexibility and the ability of muscle to burn fat? *Exercise, of course!*

Weight loss helps reverse insulin resistance and makes muscle more metabolically flexible with regard to its ability to *burn glucose.* However, even substantial weight loss (around 100 pounds) does not enhance *fat burning* per se. Exercise, on the other hand, is proven to restore the capacity of muscle mitochondria to burn fat, possibly through an increased expression of genes involved in fat burning as well as the creation of new mitochondria.[50] The higher fat-burning capacity of exercise-trained muscle is associated with improved metabolic flexibility and thus a lowered risk of developing metabolic diseases. Conversely, physical *in*activity triggers a state of metabolic *in*flexibility characterized by reduced fat burning in muscle. In fact, fat-burning enzymes are decreased in obesity and type 2 diabetes, disorders that are marked by metabolic inflexibility.[51] (See Chapter 7 for much more on exercise and muscle health.)

Excretion of Myokines

We generally don't think of muscle as having much in common with the thyroid, adrenal, pancreas, or other endocrine glands. (These endocrine glands synthesize and release vitally important hormones such as thyroxin, cortisol, and insulin.) But in a relatively recent discovery (1997 – 2003), muscle was likewise found to function as an endocrine organ. Muscle produces hundreds of signaling molecules (hormones) called "myokines"—"myo" means muscle—that exert effects within the muscle itself while also being released into the bloodstream to signal beneficial effects in other organs such as the liver, heart, brain, adipose (fat) tissue, skin, and bone. That is to say, muscle does not "crosstalk" (communicate) with other organs and tissues solely via the nervous system.[52]

Since myokines are primarily generated and released in response to muscle contraction, convincing evidence suggests that they play a key role in mediating the health-enhancing effects of exercise with respect to maintaining optimal health and preventing major chronic diseases (i.e., type 2 diabetes and metabolic syndrome). For example, specific myokines facilitate crosstalk between muscle and fat tissue that may partly account for the exercise-induced improvement in metabolic health in the obese. Myokines also contribute to exercise-induced improvements in skin aging.[5]

In a review of 55 published papers related to myokines, most of them show that exercise-induced myokines improve metabolic impairment in patients with various metabolic diseases (see chart below showing percentage of studies per disease).[53]

Classification of diseases related to myokines

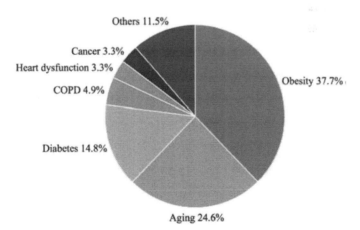

Source: Reprinted with permission from Jun Seok Son, Song Ah Chae, Eric D. Testroet, Min Du & Hyung-pil Jun (2018) Exercise-induced myokines: a brief review of controversial issues of this decade, Expert Review of Endocrinology & Metabolism, 13:1, 51-58, DOI: 10.1080/17446651.2018.1416290

Interleukin 6: The Prototype

Having been studied the most extensively among the more than 650 myokines, interleukin 6 (IL-6) is the prototype myokine. Baseline concentrations of IL-6 in the circulation can dramatically increase up to a *hundredfold* following exercise, depending on the duration and intensity of the exercise.[54] Some important health benefits of exercise have been assigned to the exercise-induced release of IL-6, which was originally referred to as the "exercise factor." These include loss of body fat and fat within muscle fibers, anti-inflammatory effects, suppression of tumor growth, appetite inhibition, and increased muscle mass and strength in response to resistance training. Furthermore, IL-6 also features a very familiar benefit: improved **blood sugar control.** IL-6 achieves this through increased glucose uptake, improved insulin action, and enhanced glucose production in the liver.[52] (see illustration below)

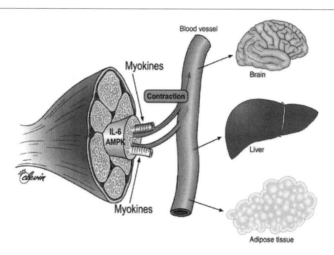

Pedersen B.K. *Muscles and Their Myokines. J. Exp. Biol. 2011;214:337–346.*

In response to muscle contraction, muscle fibers produce the myokine IL-6. IL-6 then exerts effects locally within muscle fibers. e.g., via activation of the protein AMPK – a master energy sensor that lowers blood glucose and promotes burning of stored fat (see

Chapter 7 for more on AMPK). It can also be released into the
circulation and subsequently impact distant organs and tissues.

Interestingly, pre-exercise depletion of glycogen (carbohydrate) stores accelerates the exercise-induced surge of IL-6.[55] On the other hand, carbohydrate ingestion *during* exercise lessens the IL-6 response.[52] These observations lend support to the practice of "exercising on empty" (see Chapter 11), which is also in keeping with our ancestors' ancient task of hunting wild animals under conditions of famine.

What is especially intriguing about IL-6 is that—in addition to its anti-inflammatory properties—this multifaceted molecule paradoxically also triggers pro-inflammatory reactions. One possible reason for this dichotomy is that IL-6 is not only produced in muscle tissue but in adipose (fat) tissue as well. The muscle-derived IL-6 triggered by exercise is released as an acute spike that then rapidly decreases toward pre-exercise concentrations.[56] This *short-lived and intermittent* elevation of IL-6 levels is a normal and healthy occurrence; it is responsible for the numerous health benefits previously described. In contrast, IL-6 generated by fat tissue exerts pro-inflammatory effects and is known to be *chronically elevated* in disorders associated with insulin resistance, such as metabolic syndrome, obesity, type 2 diabetes, and cardiovascular disease. Chronically high circulating levels of IL-6 are observed in people who are physically inactive, whereas low IL-6 levels are common in people who exercise regularly.[55,57]

Myostatin: The "Inverse" Myokine

Not all muscle-derived myokines are desirable. Myostatin appears to have the greatest impact on muscle mass and body fat content, but in an *inverse* manner. In other words, myostatin impairs muscle synthesis and promotes muscle breakdown while also increasing fat mass. Mutations in the myostatin gene that causes decreased myostatin production result in significantly increased muscle mass and strength; conversely, overproduction of myostatin leads to muscle atrophy.[58,59] From an evolutionary angle, why would we have evolved what seems to be a counterproductive function of muscle? Remarkably, it has been suggested that myostatin may have served as a safeguard mechanism to restrict the accumulation of muscle—a high-energy-consuming tissue—over and above essential needs.[56]

Levels of myostatin increase with advancing age and positively correlate with the development of sarcopenia, the progressive age-related decline in muscle mass and strength. Suppressing myostatin may be a promising strategy for the treatment of sarcopenia.[60] At present, it's well-documented that exercise is the most effective intervention for sarcopenia—a review of the current evidence suggests that muscle-derived myokines contribute to the beneficial effects of exercise.[59] While exercise causes an acute *increase* in IL-6 that then boosts muscle growth, both aerobic and resistance training cause a *reduction* in myostatin to prevent muscle loss. Obesity, type 2 diabetes, and metabolic syndrome—all disorders that improve with exercise—are also linked to high myostatin levels.

BDNF: "Miracle Gro" for the Brain

Cognitive impairment and dementia are serious public health threats that afflict millions of people worldwide. Tools to prevent these illnesses are critical in the effort to conquer these global epidemics that are related to aging populations. In this regard, regular exercise is front and center as an effective way to protect against cognitive decline and neurodegenerative diseases, even if people begin exercising after their midlife point. An important myokine known as brain-derived neurotrophic factor (BDNF) is partly responsible for the favorable effects of exercise on cognitive ability as well as depression and anxiety. As a myokine, BDNF is produced by muscle—although, as its name implies, it's mostly made in the brain—and is significantly increased through exercise.

For a long time, it was thought that the brain could not grow new neurons (nerve cells). However, we now know that BDNF regulates the survival, growth, repair, and maintenance of neurons. It also strengthens what's called "synaptic plasticity," which is the ability of neuronal connections (synapses, or gaps between nerve cells) to adapt or remodel themselves in response to changing conditions in the environment. This is fundamental to learning and memory. Decreased levels of BDNF accompany the neuronal dysfunction and degeneration found in many neurological diseases, such as Alzheimer's disease, Parkinson's disease, and Huntington's disease.[61]

Some studies have indicated that muscle-derived BDNF is not released into the circulation to interact with the brain, suggesting that exercise improves cognition primarily via BDNF produced in the brain.[52,59] Regardless, BDNF from muscle may still contribute to neurological benefits indirectly through the action of "intermediary" myokines. Systemic levels of two muscle-derived myokines, cathepsin B and irisin, are elevated by exercise. These myokines in turn cross the blood-brain barrier to induce production of BDNF in the brain and stimulate the formation of new neurons.[52]

In addition to its vital contributions to nerve and brain health, muscle BDNF is involved in the regeneration of damaged muscles post-exercise. BDNF from muscle has been shown to play a prominent role in the activation of muscle satellite cells (precursor stem cells) and their differentiation (conversion) into muscle fibers. Muscle BDNF is also an essential regulator of energy metabolism. The post-exercise increase in muscle BDNF production enhances fat burning in muscle and promotes mitochondrial biogenesis, which is the creation of new energy-producing mito-chondria. Conversely, insufficient production of BDNF in muscle may lead to the development of metabolic inflexibility, obesity, insulin resistance, and type 2 diabetes. ***Once again, we have a link between muscle and blood sugar control.***[56,62] Finally, muscle BDNF stimulates bone formation by inducing mineralization and the proliferation of osteoblasts (bone-forming cells).[58]

PART II

What Causes Muscle Loss?

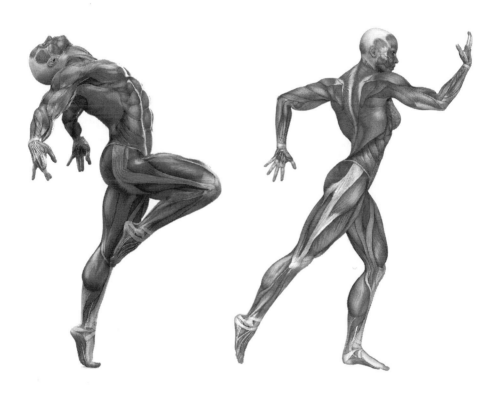

Chapter 3

Physical Inactivity

In the fifth century, the Greek physician Hippocrates wrote[1]:

"All parts of the body, if used in moderation and exercised in labors to which each is accustomed, become thereby healthy and well developed and age slowly; but if they are unused and left idle, they become liable to disease, defective in growth, and age quickly."

Hippocrates' words most certainly apply to our muscles! While many factors underlie age-related loss of muscle mass and strength, a lack of physical activity and exercise is the most important determinant.[2] Since the emergence of powered machinery, there has been about a 50% – 70% decline in people's estimated daily step numbers (see table below).[3]

Estimated Historical Reductions in Daily Steps Taken by Humans

Population	Year	Steps per day (men)	Steps per day (women)
Paleolithic	(roughly 20,000 BCE)	13,200 – 21,120	10,560
Amish	(2002)	18,425	14,196
Mean of 26 studies	(1966 – 2007)	n/a	7,473
Colorado	(2002)	6,733	6,384
U.S. adults	(2010)	5,340	4,912

Reproduced with permission from Booth FW, Roberts CK, Laye MJ. Lack of exercise is a major cause of chronic diseases. *Compr Physiol* : 1143–1211, 2012. doi:10.1002/cphy.c110025

The frequency of physical activity and muscle use declines with advancing age, potentially leading to sarcopenia (see Chapter 1). Even brief periods of reduced activity due to illness or hospitalization can accelerate the progressive loss of muscle mass with age. For example, older adults who lowered their daily step count by 76% (a mean of just 1,413 steps per day) for 14 days experienced a significant loss of leg muscle (approximately 4%) along with gains in abdominal fat. Even younger individuals in their mid-twenties lost the same percentage of leg muscle mass after reducing their daily step count by about 80% for 14 days. *However, it is important to recognize that the ability to fully recover lost muscle mass and function following periods of muscle disuse appears to be greatly diminished in older adults compared with the young.*[4]

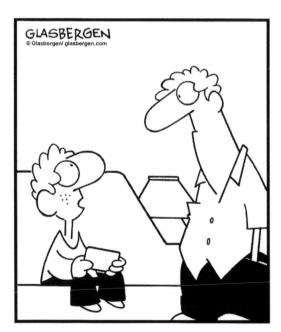

"If inactivity is bad for you, how come trees live hundreds of years?"

In order to survive, our early hunter-gatherer ancestors needed to be very physically active, walking long distances and occasionally sprinting to find food and escape predators. Most of our genes were likely programmed during this era of compulsory physical activity in a hunter-gatherer environment. In other words, exercise is built into our DNA. Our physiology has evolved to adapt to this highly physically active lifestyle, and our health has even come to rely on it.

Though today we have the same ancient genes, a sedentary environment can alter the *expression* of those genes. **The health-damaging effects of physical inactivity are comparable to the damaging effects of smoking and obesity.** In contrast, daily physical activity normalizes the expression of our genes to resemble the genetic blueprint that was designed for our survival during the Late Paleolithic era.[5,6] Let's look at how exactly inactivity causes muscle loss.

Reduced Muscle Protein Synthesis

Excluding water, muscle is made up of approximately 80% protein. Muscle proteins make up 50% – 75% of all body proteins and are constantly turning over.[7] How well we maintain our muscle mass is governed by the balance between our muscle proteins being synthesized and our muscle proteins being broken down. Resistance exercise, amino acids, and insulin are the major triggers of muscle protein synthesis (MPS). Muscle protein synthesis occurs when dietary proteins are broken down via digestion to essential amino acids that are then used to assemble new proteins that are taken up by muscle tissue.[8] Thus, among the main triggers of MPS, *only* amino acids are mandatory.

Recurrent periods of reduced physical activity cause a blunting of the MPS response to the anabolic (growth-promoting) effects of dietary protein and insulin. Decreased MPS can lead to a net negative protein balance (i.e., greater protein breakdown than synthesis), which can undermine muscle upkeep. Over the long term, it appears that muscle disuse resulting from *chronic* inactivity (which is more long term than *recurrent* inactivity) reduces the sensitivity of muscle to the anabolic stimulation of amino acids and insulin. This "anabolic resistance" may contribute to the loss of muscle mass, strength, and functionality (see Chapter 6 for more on age-related anabolic resistance). Fortunately, exercise and nutrition interventions can overcome anabolic resistance[8] (see Part III).

Insulin Resistance

Physical inactivity is also a major promoter of insulin resistance – a major contributor to sarcopenia. In just one day of sitting and lying down without any walking, the ability of younger adults to clear excess glucose from their bloodstream (signaled by insulin) decreased by at least 18%. In a less drastic restriction on activity levels, a reduction in daily steps to fewer than 4,000 steps over 1 week in a group of young men resulted in a nearly *twofold* increase in insulin resistance.[8]

So how exactly does insulin resistance affect the loss of muscle mass?

While anabolic resistance to insulin (and reduced MPS) is linked directly to muscle disuse, it's also associated with being insulin-resistant. For example, compared with healthy young adults, obese young adults with insulin resistance have been shown to exhibit blunted rates of muscle protein synthesis.[4] Insulin stimulates blood flow and perfusion into muscle tissue, thus facilitating the delivery of amino acids to muscle for MPS. When people are insulin-resistant, however, their blood vessels become unresponsive to the actions of insulin. This results in a diminished nutrient flow to muscle cells, blunted MPS, and potentially accelerated muscle atrophy.[9]

Inflammation and Oxidative Stress—Again!

While the link between physical inactivity and muscle atrophy is rather obvious, it may come as a surprise that simply being less physically active can ramp up systemic inflammation and oxidative stress. Both of these destructive processes play major roles in aging as well as the development of many age-related diseases such as cancer and cardiovascular diseases (as noted in Chapter 2). *At the genetic level, inactivity drives the expression of genes that promote the development of 35 chronic diseases.* These same genes—and the proteins they produce—are involved in pro-inflammatory signaling and oxidative stress.[10]

In studies of older adults, circulating markers of inflammation – tumor necrosis factor alpha (TNF-α) and C-reactive protein (CRP) - were increased after 2 weeks of limited walking.[4] Chronic low-grade inflammation (as commonly observed in inactivity, aging, and chronic diseases) causes tissue damage and muscle loss. Similarly, increased oxidative stress can lead to early degeneration of muscle, such as what is observed in muscular dystrophy. For example, mice genetically altered to have impaired antioxidant capacity develop significant damage and atrophy of muscle tissue that resembles myopathy (muscle disease). Both elevated inflammation levels and increased oxidative stress are key contributors to insulin resistance. Because of that, they exert an indirect effect on muscle wasting as well.[10] Since insulin resistance is essentially an intolerance to carbohydrates, could a high-carbohydrate diet possibly have adverse effects on muscle? In the next chapter, we'll explore this question in more detail.

All in all, the negative consequences of physical inactivity can be conveniently and comprehensively illustrated by the following figure:

Physical Inactivity Increases 35 Chronic Diseases

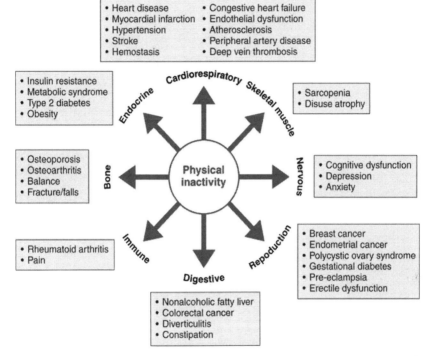

Source: Reprinted from Booth FW, Roberts CK, Thyfault JP, Ruegsegger GN, Toedebusch RG. Role of Inactivity in Chronic Diseases: Evolutionary Insight and Pathophysiological Mechanisms. Physiol Rev. 2017 Oct 1;97(4):1351-1402. doi: 10.1152/physrev.00019.2016.

Enough said?

Chapter 4

High-Carbohydrate Diets

Before we explore how a high-carbohydrate diet may tie in with muscle loss, we need to first clearly define what a "high-carbohydrate" diet is. Currently, Americans get roughly half of their calories from carbohydrates.[1] This pretty much falls in line with government recommendations: the 2015 – 2020 Dietary Guidelines for Americans jointly issued by the U.S. Department of Agriculture (USDA) and Health and Human Services (HHS) recommends that carbohydrates should make up 45% – 65% of our total daily calories.[2]

So then is a diet wherein 50% of daily calories come from carbohydrates considered to be a "high-carbohydrate" diet?

There's no clear consensus on or standardized definition of what a "high-carbohydrate" diet is. "High-carbohydrate" is a relative term.[3] In the context of this chapter, it would be more appropriate to compare *higher* to *lower* (as well as *very low*) carbohydrate diets to each other. In keeping with research studies, a "lower-carbohydrate" diet can be defined as one wherein a person consumes fewer than 25% – 30% of their total calories in the form of carbohydrates, while a *very* low-carbohydrate diet (i.e., a ketogenic one) consists of only 5% – 10% of calories coming from carbohydrates. Therefore, the current government-recommended intake of greater than 45% of total daily calories coming from carbohydrates is clearly a *higher-carbohydrate diet.*[4]

When discussing the quantity of dietary carbohydrates, it's also important to consider the *type*—that is, the *quality*—of the carbohydrates. The quality of a carbohydrate-rich food is determined by its glycemic index (GI) and its glycemic load (GL). The glycemic index is a measure of how fast a specific food raises blood glucose after consumption, whereas the glycemic load is equal to the GI multiplied by the amount of carbohydrates in a typical serving. (Remember, unlike proteins and fats, carbohydrates *directly* increase blood glucose.) The glycemic load is more practical since it reflects the glycemic response of foods as they are actually consumed. Thus, the GL is the best predictor of after-meal glucose levels. Processed carbohydrate foods such as refined grains are digested quickly and have a high GL, whereas minimally processed or unprocessed foods (e.g., berries, yams) have a moderate or low GI.[5]

Dietary Carbohydrates and Chronic Disease

Here's the eye-opener: we don't actually need to consume *any* dietary carbohydrates to survive. Surprised? Yes, that is indeed correct! While there are essential proteins and fats, **there are no essential dietary carbohydrates**.[5] The Recommended Dietary Allowance for carbohydrates is at least 130 grams per day. However, this figure represents the minimum amount of *glucose* and *not* dietary carbohydrates that we need to maintain the functioning of our brain and our nervous system. The brain and some other tissues are dependent on glucose. However, glucose can be synthesized in the liver from non-carbohydrate precursors (e.g., amino acids) when a diet includes little or no carbohydrates.[6]

Researchers have estimated the average amount of carbohydrates consumed by our Paleolithic ancestors—who lived 2.5 million to 10,000 years ago, the time when our genome evolved—to have been approximately 35% – 40% of their total calories. This estimate is based on historically studied hunter-gatherer populations. However, the diets of various modern hunter-gatherers have been found to vary considerably in their carbohydrate content, ranging from about 3% to about 50% of their total energy intake. Our ancestors who settled in northern areas such as barren tundras got about 15% or fewer of their calories from carbohydrates. In fact, a number of populations have thrived without any carbohydrates at all or only small, intermittently consumed amounts. Among these peoples are the Inuit (previously referred to as Eskimos), Laplanders (northern Europeans who largely live within the Arctic Circle), and some Native Americans.[5] On the other hand, other populations have flourished with carbohydrates as their primary energy source. Nonetheless, the carbohydrate intake of about 85% of modern hunter-gatherer societies has been relatively low, registering at fewer than 35% of their total calories, which is significantly lower than the amounts presently consumed by Americans and what's recommended by the USDA and HHS.[7] Only 14% of hunter-gatherer communities consumed half of their calories from plants.[8]

So what are the health implications of eating a higher-carbohydrate diet?

The bulk of evidence suggests that a greater reliance on animal foods paired with the low-carb consumption characteristic of hunter-gatherer societies more effectively meets human energy and nutrient requirements than a carbohydrate-centric diet does.[9] The traditional Alaskan Inuit are one of the healthiest populations in the world, with very low incidences of cardiovascular diseases despite a diet that includes few vegetables and one that's virtually devoid of carbohydrates.[10] Many other hunter-gatherer populations who subsisted on diets relatively low in carbohydrates have been shown to have been generally free of nutrition-related "diseases of civilization," such as obesity, type 2 diabetes, and coronary heart disease.[11,12]

The advent of the Neolithic Agricultural Revolution about 10,000 years ago initiated a major shift in human nutrition—we abandoned hunting/gathering diets dominated by animal products and embraced plant-based diets that were (and are) associated with a considerable increase in carbohydrate intake.[5] According to archaeological studies of Neolithic people, vitamin and mineral deficiencies resulting from this huge dietary shift likely contributed to a marked decrease in mean height. The height of male hunter-gatherers was about 5'9," while females were about 5'5" tall. However, these heights diminished to about 5'3" and 5' respectively by 3000 BCE. Consumption of fewer animal products and more plant foods has also been linked to a gradual shrinkage of the human brain, higher rates of dental caries, and a shortened life expectancy.[9]

On the other hand, in our present-day world, less-Westernized agriculturist societies such as the Kitavans (the indigenous people of Papua New Guinea) who consume a traditional diet characterized by a high carbohydrate intake along the range of 70% of their total calories are also free of those "diseases of civilization." All of these traditional diets have a key attribute in common: *carbohydrate quality*. The carbohydrate calories within these diets are largely derived from unprocessed, high-fiber plant foods (e.g., root vegetables) with low to moderate glycemic index (GI) values. By comparison, high-GI foods like refined sugars and grains contributes substantially to the total calories consumed in the typical U.S. diet. Consumption of these processed foods among non-Westernized populations such as the Kitavans is virtually nil.[13]

Ultimately, the *quality* of dietary carbohydrates appears to have a greater impact on our health and our risk of chronic diseases than the sheer *amount* of carbohydrates we consume. Diets rich in high-GL foods (e.g., refined grains, potato products, sugary beverages) are causally related to metabolic diseases such as obesity, type 2 diabetes, cardiovascular disease, and some cancers.

Conversely, non-starchy vegetables, whole fruits, legumes, and whole grains appear to exert protective effects against disease.

That said, individuals vary widely in terms of how they respond to high-GI carbohydrates. In particular, obese individuals and those with insulin resistance or diabetes typically respond poorly to high-GI-carbohydrate foods, especially if those same people are physically inactive. On the flip side, healthy people who are habitually physically active may tolerate high-GI carbohydrates without adverse metabolic effects.[5]

Nevertheless, the carbohydrate *amount* has major health implications as well. People living in Blue Zones such as Okinawa and Sardinia consume a high-carbohydrate diet and are renowned for their vitality and extreme longevity.[14] But on the other hand, the landmark PURE study conducted in 18 countries concluded that a high-carbohydrate intake increases the risk of dying.[15] It's important to point out that findings from said studies suggest associations and do not prove causation. Observational nutrition studies typically utilize food frequency questionnaires and are often confounded by bias, particularly the "healthy-user bias." That means that participants who are health-conscious are likely to engage in other healthy lifestyles that may significantly influence the outcomes of the study—they may exercise more, be less likely to smoke, manage their stress better, etc. Randomized clinical trials or RCTs, in contrast, are interventional studies that reduce much of the bias linked to observational studies. RTCs are considered to be the gold standard for investigating causal relationships and generating reliable evidence.[16] (we'll revisit the twists and turns of research studies in Chapter 8)

Increasing evidence from RTCs suggests that low-carbohydrate diets significantly improve most cardiovascular risk factors. In particular, they have been shown to lower blood pressure, triglycerides (blood fats), and inflammatory markers while simultaneously elevating levels of beneficial HDL.[17-20] Meta-analyses that combined data from multiple studies of clinical trials indicate that low-carbohydrate diets are almost always shown to be superior to other diets (usually low-fat diets) with respect to promoting weight loss.[21,22] A low-carb diet is particularly beneficial for people with type 2 diabetes.

A 2018 joint position statement from the American Diabetes Association (ADA) and the European Association for the Study of Diabetes (EASD) includes approving low-carbohydrate diets as being a safe and effective management of type 2 diabetes in adults. According to the consensus report, "Low-carbohydrate diets (26% of total energy) produce substantial reductions in HbA1c [hemoglobin A1c] at 3 months and 6 months, with diminishing effects at 12 and 24 months; no benefit of moderate carbohydrate restriction (26 – 45%) was observed."[23]

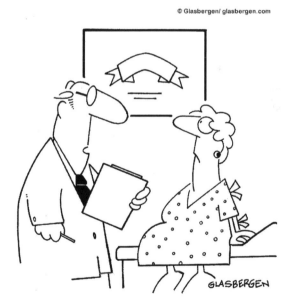

© Glasbergen/ glasbergen.com

"The high-carb diet I put you on 20 years ago gave you diabetes, high blood pressure and heart disease. Oops."

But how does carbohydrate intake relate to muscle loss?

Dietary Carbohydrates and Muscle Loss

The best way to understand the impact of carbohydrates on muscle health is to also think about the associated protein intake of that particular diet. Different carbohydrate-to-protein ratios trigger different metabolic responses in the body. Direct comparisons have been made between diets with a high carbohydrate-to-protein (CHO) ratio (55% – 60% carbohydrate; 12% – 15% protein) and diets with a low carbohydrate-to-protein (PRO) ratio (35% – 40% carbohydrate; 30% – 35% protein). Loss of body weight has been shown to be similar in both groups, but the PRO diet resulted in more favorable changes in body composition. While the weight loss in the PRO groups was predominantly fat, the CHO groups saw a greater loss of muscle mass.[24,25]

The ability of the lower-carbohydrate/higher-protein diet to preserve muscle mass is related to its effect on **blood sugar control**. Once again, we see the critical link between muscle and blood sugar control. Animal studies have shown that long-term CHO diets cause a muscle-to-fat shift that impacts the disposal of excess glucose from the bloodstream. Insulin signaling in muscle becomes blunted and fat tissue (rather than muscle tissue) becomes the primary "glucose sink" to mop up surplus blood glucose, potentially resulting in increased body fat.[26] In the PRO diets, exchanging protein (or fat) for carbohydrate lessens the need for insulin-mediated glucose uptake by muscle. The requirement for insulin is thus minimized and insulin sensitivity therefore increases in muscle tissue but is reduced in fat tissue. Greater insulin sensitivity in muscle is associated with higher muscle mass relative to body size. Furthermore, animals consuming the PRO diets had significantly elevated levels of a key signaling protein that activates muscle protein synthesis while inhibiting muscle protein breakdown. This signaling protein, Akt, is stimulated by insulin and has a greater impact when a person consumes a PRO diet. Overall, both muscle protein synthesis and muscle insulin sensitivity are higher on lower-carbohydrate diets than on higher-carbohydrate diets.[26,27]

In an experimental study, the proliferation of muscle satellite cells (muscle-specific stem cells) in petri dishes was impeded by a nutrient medium (used to grow the cells) that was high in glucose. In contrast, the proliferation of muscle satellite cells was shown to be higher in an exceptionally low (read: barely detectable) glucose environment. Although stem cells—which function to replace old and dysfunctional cells—become damaged themselves over time, they are also capable of renewing themselves. The lowered glucose concentration enhanced the self-renewal of the cultured satellite cells, enabling them to better proliferate. *Muscle stem cells play a crucial role in repairing muscle injury and maintaining muscle mass.* These findings indicate that high blood sugar levels resulting from a higher-carb diet (as well as advancing age) may adversely affect the muscle repair process and promote sarcopenia. People with diabetes in particular have an increased risk of age-related muscle atrophy.[28]

Chapter 5

Imbalanced Protein Distribution

If you don't remember anything else from this chapter, remember this: *muscle can't be built without amino acids!* In addition to being building blocks for muscle protein, essential amino acids from protein foods directly stimulate muscle protein synthesis.[1] New and fascinating research from leading authorities on protein nutrition suggests that particularly in terms of meal distribution and timing, the protein intake of most American adults is inadequate for maintaining optimal muscle mass, strength, and function.[2-5]

Throughout our lives, our muscle mass is maintained by a tightly regulated balance between muscle protein synthesis (MPS) and muscle protein breakdown (MPB). Regulation of muscle mass falls under the direction of the critically important protein called "mTOR," short for "mechanistic target of rapamycin." Given its role, mTOR seems appropriately named—it brings to mind the god of thunder in Viking mythology, similarly named Thor and similarly associated with power and strength. Although mTOR is not whatsoever connected to Thor (disappointingly), mTOR does anchor a powerful signaling pathway that switches on the cellular "machinery" that the body uses to manufacture muscle protein.[6]

The optimum amount of dietary protein that adults need for general health is open to question. The current Recommended Daily Allowance for protein (0.8 grams of protein per kilogram of body weight per day, or about 0.4 grams per pound of body weight per day) represents the bare minimum needed to prevent a clear protein deficiency and sustain growth and development. The RDA for protein is a one-size-fits-all recommendation that ignores age-related changes in metabolism, immunity, and hormone levels. Based on the RDA, the recommended daily protein intake is a paltry 55 – 57 grams for men and 47 – 48 grams for women.[7]

In order to conform to the guidelines for the two other macronutrients—fat and carbohydrate—the Food and Nutrition Board also established an Acceptable Macronutrient Distribution Range (AMDR) for protein as a *percentage of calorie intake*. The AMDR for protein is 10% – 35% of total calories (for a woman on a 2,000 calorie diet, this translates to 50 – 175 grams of protein). Unlike the RDA recommendation (which again represents a minimal level of protein intake), the AMDR reflects an optimal protein intake based on studies that suggest that higher protein intakes result in health benefits and a reduced risk of chronic diseases. Interestingly, the lowest level of protein intake specified in the AMDR (10%) is higher than the RDA for protein.[8]

The amount of protein needed to optimize mTOR signaling and muscle protein synthesis should largely shape adult protein requirements. In presenting evidence-based recommendations for optimal dietary protein intake in older adults, the PROT-AGE Study Group released a consensus position paper stating that higher protein intakes well above the RDA recommendation—namely, a *minimum* of 1.0 to 1.2 grams per kilogram of body weight per day, or about 0.5 grams per pound of body weight per day—may be needed for optimal health in many adults aged 65 years and older, **particularly for the growth and maintenance of muscle.** Even higher protein intakes of *more* than 1.2 g/kg of body weight/day are suggested for older adults who exercise and are otherwise active (protein turnover, or renewal, is accelerated with exercise). But rather than expressing protein needs as a simple percentage of overall daily calorie intake, the position paper emphasizes the importance of the quantity and quality of the protein (or amino acids) consumed during individual meals, pointing out that this is what's needed to maximize muscle protein synthesis. This concept of a "meal threshold" is physiologically important to preserve muscle mass and function.[4]

Among the essential amino acids we need to obtain from our diet, *leucine* has a unique role. That's because the amount of dietary protein at a meal needed to trigger mTOR and MPS is dependent on the meal's leucine content. Clinical trials indicate that meals containing more than 2.2 grams of leucine are required to activate mTOR signaling; conversely, meals with fewer than 1.8 grams of leucine have no effect on mTOR.[2]

So what does this mean in terms of daily *protein* intake for adults?

A meal threshold of at least 30 grams of protein (e.g., a 3.5-ounce chicken breast) fully stimulates muscle protein synthesis.[3] Consuming about 30 grams of high-quality protein per meal provides about 2.5 grams of leucine,[9] which is more than enough to turn on mTOR signaling and MPS. While many American adults may consume enough total protein throughout their day, the typical pattern of ingesting more than 60% of their daily protein allotment during the evening meal and less than 15% at breakfast is not favorable for maximizing muscle health.[2] When compared with the conventional practice of consuming most of their daily protein intake during their evening meal, the rate of muscle protein synthesis in healthy adults was reported to be 25% higher when the same amount of protein was evenly distributed in an amount of roughly 30 grams consumed across breakfast, lunch, and dinner.[10] To the contrary, in children and young adults, high levels of anabolic hormones (e.g., insulin, IGF-1, and growth hormone) compensate for uneven protein distribution by enabling more efficient use of protein for muscle health.[3] Thus, when youth eat a donut for breakfast, a peanut-butter-and-jelly sandwich for lunch, and a hamburger for dinner, their growth is not impeded.

A protein intake of *30 – 50 grams* at each of the three daily meals is ideal for optimizing muscle health as well as improving other metabolic functions of protein such as appetite control, blood sugar control, and metabolic rate.[9] Protein consumption of only about 15 grams (represented by a breakfast of two eggs) produces little or no *anabolic stimulus* to muscle, although it does contribute to total daily protein consumption. On the other hand, protein intake in excess of 50 grams or so at a single meal is oxidized as fuel and likewise does not provide any additional anabolic stimulus to muscle. But there's a sweet spot in the middle: a 6-ounce (42 – 48 grams) serving of beef tenderloin will top out your protein allotment for dinner with regard to triggering MPS.

The per-meal range of 30 – 50 grams of dietary protein being needed to trigger mTOR is consistent with a person's protein needs expressed as a percentage of their total calorie intake. The average man consuming 2,500 calories per day to maintain his weight would require a total of roughly 125 grams of protein daily. That's based on a moderate 20% of calories from protein, which is the midpoint of the AMDR. Similarly, the average woman ingesting 2,000 daily calories needs about 100 grams of protein for optimal muscle health. *While still moderate, these more desirable values for protein requirements are more than twice the RDA!*

After a person consumes a meal containing high-quality protein, their MPS increases by about threefold and then peaks around 1.5 hours before returning to baseline rates within 2 – 3 hours. This happens despite a persistence of elevated plasma leucine levels and mTOR signaling. Thereafter, a "refractory period" sets in whereby muscle becomes resistant to leucine stimulation. This ceiling on MPS (also referred to as "muscle full") allows muscle time to recover or reset its protein-making machinery prior to the next meal.[2,11] With that in mind, we should ideally space our meals about 3 – 5 hours apart. Doing so allows us to accommodate this refractory period and maximize our MPS.[12]

As you may have noted by now, protein needs can be expressed in three different ways: (1) on a per-meal basis, (2) as a percentage of calorie intake (AMDR), and (3) as grams per kilogram of body weight per day. While the AMDR for protein is valuable for justifying the need for higher protein intakes to prevent chronic diseases, adult protein requirements are *not* proportional to total calorie intake—rather, they're proportional to body weight.[3] For example, using the AMDR method, when calories are reduced in an effort to lose weight, protein intake would unfavorably decline as well. If the average woman who normally consumes 2,000 daily calories decides to begin a 1,200-calorie weight-loss diet, she would cut critical protein intake by 40%! (Assuming that she gets 20% of her calories from protein.)

A meal-to-meal determination of protein needs is an innovative, convenient, and effective strategy that's based on the quantity and quality of protein needed to simulate mTOR and MPS. Dr. Donald Layman, Professor Emeritus of Nutrition at the University of Illinois and a world-leading expert on dietary protein and amino acids, stresses the importance of the first meal and the last meal of the day. "It's important to have enough protein at your first meal to fully trigger muscle, because that's the most catabolic [breaking down tissues for energy] period of the day. You are coming off a 12-hour fast when your body degrades muscle protein to supply amino acids to the brain, liver, and other organs; at the same time, protein synthesis is low." Layman favors a person's last meal (typically dinner) being their next substantial protein meal to minimize the nighttime catabolic period. In addition, after each meal there is a refractory period of about 5 hours before the muscle system can totally reset; therefore, spreading out the major meals maximizes the effectiveness of the protein that's eaten.

"Total protein is most important—it should be at least 1.2 g/kg body weight/day up to 1.8 g/kg body weight/day [or topping out close to 1 gram per pound of body weight per day]. Your first and last meal should probably each exceed 40 grams of protein to maximize the anabolic effect in muscle; distribution of any additional protein beyond breakfast and dinner doesn't make much difference," says Layman. Otherwise stated, consuming about 30 grams of protein within 5 hours after the first meal or last meal does *not* trigger mTOR since it has already been stimulated and will run for at least 5 hours. Thus, any amount of protein you ingest at lunch will contribute to total daily protein but there is no evidence that the lunch meal will stimulate muscle protein synthesis. Nonetheless, a midday meal containing at least 30 grams of protein is important for stabilizing blood sugar levels, providing satiety, and boosting metabolism.

The anabolic effect of protein and the quantity required to trigger muscle protein synthesis varies with age, with older adults needing a greater protein intake than younger individuals (see the PROT-AGE Study Group determination). Once individuals hit age 30 or thereabouts, the anabolic effects of growth hormones (e.g., insulin, growth hormone, IGF-1, and steroid hormones) that are pronounced in children and young adults begin to significantly wane. Incidentally, these hormonal effects explain how young athletes can boast about huge muscle gains on a substandard vegan diet of lower-quality protein. Case in point: gains in muscle mass and strength did not differ between resistance-trained young men (roughly 26 years of age) who consumed a high-protein, plant-based diet versus a protein-matched omnivorous diet.[13]

As we age and our anabolic hormones become essentially ineffective at activating MPS, exercise and diet *quality* become the limiting factors for promoting and sustaining optimal muscle health. The muscle protein synthesis response to a meal decreases throughout our adult lives, a phenomenon that's referred to as "anabolic resistance." (We'll get much more into this in the next chapter.)

Dietary Protein and Exercise Recovery

When protein consumption is combined with resistance exercise, a synergistic effect on muscle protein synthesis occurs. Resistance training lowers the threshold at which dietary protein activates mTOR. In other words, exercise sensitizes muscle to the anabolic effects of protein, and this heightened sensitivity continues for at least 24 hours after a workout. Possible mechanisms for this effect include an increased uptake and sensing of amino acids within the muscle cell as well as enhanced insulin sensitivity. Though saying "sensitized muscle" implies that less protein is needed after training to trigger muscle, a higher protein intake may nevertheless be necessary to maximize MPS owing to the greater exercise-induced capacity to utilize amino acids. Without any protein intake (e.g., after an overnight fast), resistance exercise causes more muscle protein degradation than synthesis, resulting in a net breakdown of muscle protein. By considerably boosting MPS relative to MPB, protein consumption leads to a positive net balance in muscle protein.[2] That is to say, resistance training drives muscle growth *provided that* sufficient protein is accessible at the time. I'll repeat: ***you can't build muscle without amino acids, a.k.a. protein!***

The greatest muscle benefits are achieved when a meal rich in protein is consumed *after* exercise. That's because muscles are more responsive to amino acids at this time. During the post-exercise recovery period, depending on the exerciser's age, the general consensus says that it's best to consume 20 – 40 grams of high-quality animal protein to maximize muscle protein synthesis. This protein dose provides sufficient *leucine* (about 1.8 – 4.0 grams) to trigger post-exercise MPS.[14] Whey protein is the ideal post-workout food based on its superior anabolic properties, i.e., rapid digestion and rich leucine content.[15] Protein should preferably be consumed within 2 hours of having completed exercising. That said, exactly when people should eat their post-workout protein meal is influenced by their training status and when they ate their pre-exercise protein meal (or didn't).[2,16]

Timing of Post-Exercise Protein

People who are physically inactive (untrained) are generally in a catabolic state with regard to muscle—they're breaking down more muscle protein than they're synthesizing, resulting in a net negative protein balance. When these individuals begin an exercise program (particularly resistance training), MPS surges and persists for at least 24 hours after exercise. In other words, they have much room for improvement. (In a similar manner, heavier people lose weight more rapidly and for a longer time when restricting calories.) Therefore, protein consumed immediately—as in fewer than 2 hours post-exercise—may be especially valuable as a means to reverse catabolism and enhance exercise-induced activation of both mTOR and MPS in *untrained* individuals.

On the other hand, with progressive training, the MPS response is adaptively reduced and returns to pre-exercise levels more rapidly. Thus, protein ingestion during the immediate post-exercise period may be comparatively less important in *trained* individuals, meaning that essentially, regular training leaves less room for improvement, a concept known as the "law of diminishing returns." Nevertheless, due to the short-lived MPS response in trained individuals, it may still be important for them to immediately replenish their protein to optimize their MPS.[14,16]

Resistance exercise in a fasted state—for example, following an overnight fast—causes a "doubling down" effect on muscle protein catabolism (breakdown) and a prolonged net negative protein balance that is *not* offset by exercise-induced increases in MPS. In this circumstance, it's an advantage to halt the catabolic process and shift to an anabolic state by consuming high-quality protein immediately after exercising. In contrast, consuming high-quality protein *before* a workout enables amino acid delivery to muscle that's sustained far into the recovery period, thereby making it less necessary to immediately consume post-exercise protein. However, if an individual eats their pre-exercise protein meal more than 3 – 4 hours before they exercise, then they still benefit from immediately consuming protein post-workout (refer back to the previously discussed refractory period).[16]

Muscle Genes and Muscle Performance/Recovery

While the proper timing and distribution of protein doses throughout the day is an effective strategy, an individual's *total daily protein intake* (ideally, think in the neighborhood of 1 gram per pound of body weight per day) remains the most important determinant of the ability of protein to promote muscle growth and strength during resistance training. Some have argued that eating a balanced diet—one with sufficient protein and calories—in tandem with doing resistance exercises may be all you need to do to support muscle health and drive muscle growth. In other words, they say that the addition of a post-workout protein shake is redundant.[12] However, it may be necessary to consume a large amount of protein immediately after a workout to markedly enhance and prolong the expression of key anabolic and anti-catabolic genes. Specifically, in a study in young, healthy trained males, the consumption of 40 grams of whey protein compared with consumption of moderate-to-small quantities of 10 – 20 grams of whey protein after resistance exercise was shown to increase the production of amino acid transporters that facilitate the entry of amino acids into the muscle cell. Amino acid transporters are also linked to mTOR signaling. In this same study, the much larger protein dose also blunted the expression of a gene related to the degradation of muscle proteins. *Importantly, these effects on gene expression occurred when the protein was given immediately after the subjects completed exercising; these effects were absent when they consumed a second portion of protein 6 hours later.*[17] Thus, substantial protein intake during the early post-exercise recovery period appears to trigger genes that regulate muscle growth and maintenance.

Beyond muscle enhancement, immediate post-workout protein consumption has been shown to improve exercise-induced training adaptations related to muscle performance and recovery. Evidence from systematic reviews of mostly RCTs supports the ergogenic (performance-enhancing) potential of whey protein and its ability to accelerate the recovery of muscle function following resistance exercise.[18,19] Post-exercise whey protein consumption also lowers blood levels of myoglobin and creatine kinase, which are biomarkers of muscle damage and

Whey Protein Alternatives

If you are allergic to dairy, you are most likely reacting to the casein component rather than the whey fraction, which is much less allergenic. Nevertheless, other good options are goat whey protein and egg, beef, or pea protein powders. Also, you may better tolerate a hydrolyzed (partially digested) whey powder. If you cannot eat dairy due to lactose intolerance, choose whey protein *isolate* over whey *concentrate*. Keep in mind, however, that whey is truly a super food with "bonus" properties that include immune-enhancing factors. Your best alternative to cow whey protein is goat whey protein.

inflammation induced by exercise. Furthermore, the high concentration of branched-chain amino acids in whey protein provides a source of energy to fuel muscles and delay the onset of fatigue, thus improving exercise performance and reducing the risk of injuries.

Older Adults Need More Protein

Older adults apparently require higher intakes of post-exercise protein in order to maximize their anabolic response to training. In *young adults*, the amount of post-exercise dietary protein needed to activate MPS above exercise alone begins at 5 grams and plateaus at 20 grams. No further protein synthesis occurs with higher-protein intakes. (However, as previously noted, even young adults apparently may need much a higher amount of post-workout whey protein to favorably affect the expression of muscle genes.) In contrast, in *older adults*, ingestion of 40 grams of whey protein has been shown to elevate MPS to a greater degree than ingestion of only 20 grams of whey protein. Since the muscle-building effect of resistance exercise is blunted in aged muscle (see next chapter), older adults who consume a relatively high amount of whey protein of around 40 grams after exercising may potentially boost their rates of MPS to be what young adults experience.[20]

Rest Days

It's clear that protein consumption after resistance training promotes muscle growth. Surprisingly, however, consuming enough high-quality protein with each meal may actually be more important for muscle maintenance when you're *not* training. Dietary protein can provide the stimulus for mTOR activation and muscle protein synthesis that's missing on rest days.[21] In fact, *more* leucine-rich protein may be needed on rest days compared with workout days to maximize and/or sustain MPS.[14] (This is not welcoming news for vegans.)

So what about those carbs? And glycogen?

Carbohydrates and Glycogen

According to current dogma, ingesting carbs along with protein following workouts will enhance the anabolic effect of exercise by raising insulin levels. However, the scientific evidence does not support this claim. Several studies have shown that the combined effects of carbohydrate and protein consumption after resistance exercise does *not* further increase MPS versus protein intake alone.[11,12,22] The relatively low concentrations of insulin stimulated by dietary protein is sufficient to achieve maximal increase in muscle protein synthesis and/or reduce protein breakdown, while the additional rise in insulin levels triggered by carbs does not appear to provide an even greater stimulus for protein synthesis.[22]

Not only are carbohydrates *not* needed to build muscle, they are also *not* required to fuel muscles via replenishment of muscle glycogen (the storage form of carbohydrates). When carbohydrates are not available—say, if you're pursuing a ketogenic diet or fasting—glycogen synthesis can be induced by a process called "gluconeogenesis." During gluconeogenesis, non-carbohydrate molecules such as lactate, amino acids, and glycerol (from burning fat) are used to make glucose in the liver. The "new" glucose is then transported to muscle tissue, where it's stored as glycogen.[23,24] In fact, the rate of glycogen synthesis after weightlifting *without* consuming any post-exercise calories is higher than rates reported after submaximal exercise (85% of age-adjusted maximal heart rate) *accompanied by* consuming carbohydrates during the first 6 hours of recovery.[25]

In addition, compared to endurance training, glycogen is less important for resistance work. While muscle glycogen is reduced by more than 60% after 2 hours of running,[24] high-intensity resistance workouts (6 – 9 sets per muscle group) result in only a 36 – 39% depletion of muscle glycogen.[16] Furthermore, these intense resistance training sessions require a long recovery period, thus allowing plenty of time to replenish muscle glycogen stores for the next workout. In any case, a post-workout drink of whey protein (a.k.a. amino acids) along with exercise-induced lactate may be sufficient to restock muscle glycogen via gluconeogenesis without any need for carbs.

Plant- vs. Animal-Based Proteins

Plant-based proteins are rich in fiber and micronutrients and are associated with various health benefits. However, when it comes to muscle-building potential, animal protein is clearly superior. A majority of studies have shown that animal-sourced protein is more effective than plant-sourced protein at building and sustaining muscle mass. For example, 24 grams of whey protein per day led to an increase of 3.3 kg in lean tissue (muscle) in young men after 36 weeks of resistance training, while in comparison, soy protein increased lean mass by only 1.8 kg. Another study showed that animal protein (1.7 – 40 grams) from whey, skimmed milk, or beef triggered significantly greater muscle protein synthesis in healthy adults than an equivalent amount of soy protein did. What's more, long-term consumption of a vegetarian diet among older women has been associated with decreases in muscle mass when compared to older women eating an omnivorous diet.[5]

Determining factors for assessing the quality of dietary protein include amino acid composition, protein digestibility, and protein bioavailability. The best indicator of protein quality is the Protein

Digestibility Corrected Amino Acid Score (PDCAAS). A protein with a PDCAAS score of less than 100% cannot fully satisfy the body's essential amino acid requirements. While animal proteins have a PDCAAS value of 100%, plant-sourced proteins (excepting some soy protein isolate *powders*) come in below 100%. Also, nondigestible fiber in plant foods slows down digestion. For example, the protein in whole peas (which are high in fiber) is 35% less bioavailable than the isolated and processed pea protein (which is low in fiber) used as a supplement.[26] Notably, good ol' peanut butter scores an unimpressive 45%, while wheat gluten checks in at only 25% (this has the lowest PDCAAS score).[27]

In addition to their relatively poor digestibility, plant foods (e.g., rice, wheat, corn, potatoes, vegetables, cereals, legumes, processed soy foods, nuts, and seeds) have a lower total amount and less balanced proportions of essential amino acids compared to what animal foods (e.g., meat, dairy, eggs, seafood, etc.) have. It's especially worth noting that the amino acid *leucine* plays a particularly central role as a potent anabolic signaling molecule for muscle protein synthesis and that the leucine content of plant proteins is commonly lower than that of animal proteins.[27]

Other essential amino acids are also lacking in plant proteins. Though they contain all of the essential amino acids, plant proteins have one or more deficient, or *limiting amino acids*. For example, lysine is the first limiting amino acid in wheat—it's present in the lowest amount relative to the amount needed to construct protein. ***Once a limiting amino acid in a particular protein is used up, muscle protein synthesis comes to a halt.*** All of the other amino acids in that protein will then be oxidized for energy rather than efficiently used for protein synthesis.[27] Amino acids cannot be stored in the body for later use.

As an analogy, consider a store manager planning to sell 20 baseball uniforms that each consist of a cap, shirt, pants, and socks.

The store's supplier is supposed to ship 20 of each of the components to the store but mistakenly sends only 18 caps. Consequently, the manager can only sell 18 uniforms because the shortage of caps limits what is considered to be a "full uniform." Since the store has no storage space for the extra uniform components, they're wasted.

Studies have demonstrated that amino acids derived from soy protein are broken down (to urea) to a greater extent than amino acids from dairy proteins are. That greater breakdown means the amino acids are less usable for protein synthesis in muscle and other tissues. Indeed, maintenance of muscle mass may be adversely affected by chronic and exclusive intake of plant proteins due in part to limiting amino acids such lysine in wheat and corn as well as sulfur amino acids in legumes.[27] Animal proteins, on the other hand, do not have limiting amino acids.

Because of these shortfalls, it's necessary to consume large quantities of plant proteins to achieve an anabolic effect similar to what's offered by animal protein. In an animal experiments, rats needed to eat *triple* the amount of an initial dose of wheat protein in order to attain the same rate of mTOR signaling that was observed when the rats ate a *lower* (than the initial wheat protein dose) amount of whey protein.[28] In a clinical study, neither 20 grams nor 40 grams of soy protein isolate were capable of stimulating MPS in elderly people who were in resting conditions. Compared to whey, individuals burned off substantially more of the soy protein for energy instead of using it for muscle enhancement.[29]

Nevertheless, on a global scale, plant proteins make up a greater portion of people's protein consumption than animal proteins do. What's more, older adults tend to eat fewer animal foods owing to factors such as a blunted appetite for meats, impaired chewing ability, and socioeconomic issues. But *eating high-quality protein at each meal is particularly vital for older adults* because the ability to respond to the anabolic stimulus from amino acids is impaired during aging. In light of these concerns, various strategies to enhance the anabolic potential of plant proteins are being investigated. These initiatives include fortifying plant-based proteins with specific essential amino acids (particularly leucine), blending together different plant proteins, combining plant proteins with animal proteins, and selectively breeding plants.[27]

But! Eating high quantities of plant proteins carries the disadvantage of greater carbohydrate consumption, which—when eaten in excess—drives weight (fat) gain. For example, approximately 2 grams of muscle-building leucine are provided by both a 3-ounce serving of lean beef and 2.5 cups of soybeans.[30] However, the soybeans also contribute about 140 grams of carbohydrates, whereas the beef has 0 carbs. Considering that about 75% of American adults are carb-intolerant, excessive carb consumption may contribute to the development of obesity, abnormal blood fats, and other metabolic disorders. The good news is that consumption of meat can dramatically reduce the need for carbohydrate-rich plant-based foods as a major source of essential amino acids.[5]

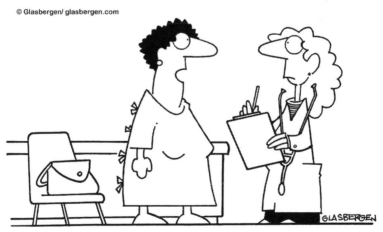

"If a vegetarian diet is good for losing weight, how come they use grain to fatten pigs and cows?"

Meat is an abundant source of important nonessential nutrients (meaning that the body can make them to some degree), including taurine, carnosine, anserine, and creatine. These nutrients are absent from plants but have critical physiological functions, particularly in anti-oxidative and anti-inflammatory reactions. Taurine, for example, is a sulfur-containing amino acid required for protecting the eyes, heart, muscle, and other tissues from oxidative damage and degradation. Carnosine is an antioxidant compound composed of two amino acids (a dipeptide) that maintains neurological, immunological, cardiovascular, and muscular functions. It also acts to buffer the increased acid that accumulates during intense exercise, thus reducing fatigue and improving exercise performance. Anserine is another dipeptide with physiological functions similar to carnosine, including acid buffering and antioxidation. Among its several roles, preformed creatine (from the diet) enables its component amino acids (arginine, glycine, and methionine) to be available for muscle protein synthesis rather than creatine synthesis.[31,32]

In general, animal foods are much more nutrient-dense than plant foods are. (That is, animal foods offer a higher quantity of micronutrients per calorie of food.) When a study evaluated the least expensive diets produced from available foods for nutritional adequacy, more nutrient deficiencies and a larger excess of calories (as well as a need to eat more food) were observed in plants-only diets.[33] The nutritional superiority of animal food over plant foods is not unexpected since we humans are composed of the same chemicals that other land-dwelling mammals are, and for the most part we require the same nutrients that they do.[34] The notion that meat is unhealthy and environmentally harmful is baseless. Unfortunately, myths claiming that a greater consumption of animal protein is harmful persist. For example, allegations that higher protein intake is damaging to kidney and bone health are completely unsubstantiated.[35] (See Chapter 8 for much more about myths linking animal protein to chronic diseases and global warming.)

Higher Dietary Protein and Weight Loss

Finally, although we already discussed this point in Chapter 4, the evidence for weight-management benefits of increased dietary protein is so robust that it bears repeating: diets composed of higher-protein/lower-carbohydrate content are superior to high-carbohydrate/low-fat/low-protein diets with regard to improving body composition and protecting muscle during weight loss. These superior diets also increase satiety and boost metabolism seeing as proteins take far more calories (20% – 30%) to process in the body than fats (0 – 3%) or carbs (5% – 10%) do.[36] Conventional higher-carbohydrate diets lead to a 30% – 40% loss of muscle, whereas higher-protein diets cut muscle loss to less than 15%. When higher-protein diets are paired with exercise, muscle loss comes to a standstill. Furthermore, long-term maintenance of weight loss is associated with the preservation of muscle (as well as bone) that is evident in people who eat diets higher in protein.[3]

Chapter 6

Anabolic Resistance

Anabolic resistance describes the blunted stimulation of muscle protein synthesis that develops in older adults in response to amino acids/protein, insulin, or exercise. Compared to young muscle, aging muscle is generally less responsive to these muscle-building triggers. Following resistance exercise and consuming amino acids, muscle protein synthesis has been shown to be delayed by about 3 hours in older men (aged approximately 70).[1]

Muscle fibers are composed of many long, threadlike strands of myofibrils that drive the contraction and relaxation of muscles. Myofibrils are composed of myofibrillar proteins, the most abundant proteins in muscle. Anabolic resistance can lead to negative net protein balance, primarily within the myofibrillar protein fraction of muscle. A negative net protein balance in which muscle protein breakdown exceeds muscle protein synthesis can result in muscle atrophy. Anabolic resistance is thus a major driver of sarcopenia, the age-related loss of muscle mass and strength.[2-5]

Anabolic resistance can also occur in younger adults after short periods of muscle disuse, such as bed rest due to injury or illness. In one study of men around 22 years old, just 5 days of leg immobilization resulted in a considerable loss (roughly 4%) of quadriceps muscle mass.[6] Specifically, the leg immobilization was found to cause a decline in the rates of MPS that was attributed to the rapid onset of anabolic resistance of muscle to amino acids derived from dietary proteins. Although the recovery of short-term losses in muscle mass and strength is quicker in younger individuals, the accumulation of such brief stretches of muscle disuse (e.g., hospitalizations of 5 – 6 days followed by a week of recovery) over a lifetime may play a major role in the development of age-related sarcopenia.

It should be noted that not all studies support the existence of anabolic resistance in healthy older adults. Two studies, for instance, concluded that aging does not suppress the anabolic response to amino acids and protein.[7,8] These inconsistent findings between studies may be explained by differences in the methodology used to assess protein synthesis, particularly the specific type of muscle protein subfraction that was analyzed.[9] Following protein consumption, resistance training primarily increases synthesis of the myofibrillar proteins. Subsequent gains in muscle mass (hypertrophy) occur when acute bouts of resistance training practiced over time result in greater synthesis than breakdown of myofibrillar protein. Rather than examining myofibrillar protein per se, some studies (including the two studies mentioned here) measured the synthesis of "mixed muscle protein," which consists of myofibrillar proteins as well as non-myofibrillar proteins such as mitochondrial protein. However, mixed protein synthesis is less responsive than myofibrillar protein per se to resistance exercise alone or in combination with amino acid consumption.[9] It is also *not* associated with muscle hypertrophy.[10]

Causes of Anabolic Resistance

As discussed in Chapter 3, periods of muscle disuse due to injury/illness or a sedentary lifestyle cause anabolic resistance by decreasing the sensitivity of muscle to the growth-stimulating effects of amino acids and insulin. At the molecular level, recurrent or chronic inactivity blunts the activation of the protein-sensing mTOR pathway.[2] Recall that mTOR is the master regulator of MPS and muscle hypertrophy. Found within all types of cells, the mTOR protein is the foundation of a signaling pathway that regulates nearly every aspect of metabolism. In particular, mTOR controls the balance between anabolism (building up) and catabolism (breaking down) in response to various nutritional and environmental cues.[11]

Signaling from mTOR must be properly balanced—both too little and too much mTOR activity can lead to muscle atrophy. When consumption of nutrients (primarily amino acids) is plentiful, activation of mTOR drives anabolic processes such as cell growth and protein synthesis while shutting down catabolic (breaking down) processes such as autophagy.[11] Autophagy (self-eating) is a quality-control mechanism whereby damaged proteins and other "expired" cell components are degraded and recycled for energy and/or the repair needs of the cell. Autophagy can be likened to a cellular "housekeeping" process designed to mop up cellular waste and maintain cell function. On that account, when calorie intake is reduced—or when an individual is fasting—mTOR signaling is suppressed and desirable autophagy is switched on.[12]

Autophagy

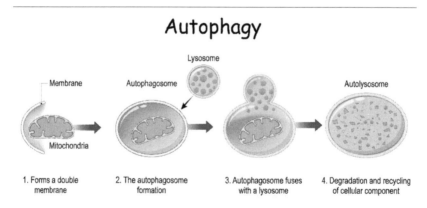

| 1. Forms a double membrane | 2. The autophagosome formation | 3. Autophagosome fuses with a lysosome | 4. Degradation and recycling of cellular component |

Autophagy begins with the formation of a double membrane around targeted cell components. In this case, those components are dysfunctional mitochondria. The double membrane then expands to form an autophagosome, which is a vesicle that engulfs the defective mitochondria. As the autophagosome fuses with another vesicle called a "lysosome," the expendable cargo is sequestered for degradation and recycling.

Autophagy is a key player with respect to the association between mTOR and muscle health. How? Autophagy preserves and increases muscle mass by removing damaged muscle fibers and regenerating new muscle fibers. At the cellular level, the ability of autophagy to recycle cellular "garbage" generates the energy that's required to stimulate the differentiation of muscle stem cells into muscle fibers.[13] However, autophagy that is not kept in check can get out of control! If excessive autophagy destroys cell components beyond a certain threshold, loss of cellular function and ultimately cell death (i.e., muscle atrophy) will occur.[14]

Age-related autophagy and muscle atrophy

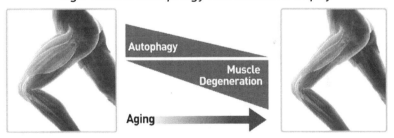

*Reprinted with permission from: Park, S.S., Y.K. Seo, and K.S. Kwon, Sarcopenia targeting with autophagy mechanism by exercise. BMB Rep, 2019. **52**(1): p. 64-69.*

In muscle, autophagy progressively declines with age, correlating with increasing muscle degeneration. Age-related muscle loss results from reductions in both the number and size of muscle fibers. Exercise suppresses this aging-induced muscle atrophy by boosting autophagy to ensure muscle maintenance.

The effect of chronic inactivity on increasing anabolic resistance and the consequent muscle loss (which happens through diminished mTOR activation) is rather easy to understand since it results in reduced muscle protein synthesis.[2] Chronic inactivity also results in excessive autophagy, which also leads to muscle loss. Therefore, over time, decreased physical activity can lead to a negative protein balance and muscle atrophy.

On the other hand, there may be a role for impaired regulation of mTOR and autophagy in the development of *age-associated* anabolic resistance. This scenario appears to be more complex. In healthy muscle, activation of mTOR is inhibited during the fasting state (e.g., overnight) while autophagy is turned on. This is critical for the upkeep of your muscles! Autophagy helps maintain what's called "proteostasis," which is a healthy balance between protein synthesis and protein degradation.[15] However, in aging or unhealthy muscle, mTOR signaling is activated rather than inhibited during fasting and remains stuck at full throttle. This sustained activation of mTOR in muscle blocks autophagy ("cellular cleanup") and leads to the buildup of abnormal or damaged proteins within the muscle cell, thereby compromising the structural integrity of muscle and resulting in muscle atrophy.[5]

It's worthwhile to compare anabolic resistance with insulin resistance in muscle seeing as they both increase with age and induce each other. In insulin resistance, the muscle cell's reduced capacity to "sense" insulin after meals - reflected in high fasting insulin levels - is linked to obesity and chronic diseases. In anabolic resistance, *abnormally* increased activation of mTOR in the fasting state impairs the ability of muscle cells to respond to amino acids after consumption of protein (due to chronic suppression of autophagy that undermines muscle integrity and function). Aging is associated with increasing levels of blood glucose and decreasing rates of MPS. Elevated levels of insulin and overactivation of mTOR in the fasting state may serve as a compensatory mechanism to maintain normal levels of blood glucose and MPS, respectively, during aging.[16] ***Studies*** *suggest the existence of an inherent defect within aging muscle that disrupts anabolic signaling. This may play a central role in the development of both insulin and anabolic resistance.*[5,16]

Not unexpectedly, obesity is also linked to anabolic resistance. Effective treatment of obesity should incorporate interventions to enhance muscle metabolism, namely high-quality protein consumption and resistance exercise. However, evidence from a study published in 2019 in the journal *Frontiers in Nutrition* indicates that the muscle in obese individuals is resistant to the anabolic actions of exercise and dietary protein consumption. Insulin resistance is a likely contributing factor, though not all individuals with obesity are insulin-resistant. Exercise combined with diet strategies that incorporate higher protein intakes of more than 1.2 g/kg body weight/day (i.e., more than 0.5 grams per pound body weight per day) are advisable (see next section).[17]

Nutrition and Exercise Strategies to Overcome Anabolic Resistance

Anabolic resistance can be counteracted by two strategies: (1) amplify the anabolic signal to construct muscle protein by eating more protein; (2) enhance the sensitivity of muscle to amino acids and insulin through increased daily physical activity and commitment to a regular exercise regimen.[18] In other words, a higher-protein diet and exercise, primarily *resistance* exercise, act synergistically to reverse the anabolic resistance to MPS that occurs during aging.

The amount of dietary protein relative to lean body mass (body weight excluding fat) needed by older adults to maximize MPS is about 140% greater than what's required by younger individuals. That's more than double! During at least two meals, older adults should consume 30 – 50 grams of high-quality protein that provides at least 3 grams or so of leucine. This will offset anabolic resistance and help maintain muscle mass during aging. However, the MPS response is blunted in both older adults who are unable to consume multiple high-protein meals and in vegans who consume lower-quality plant proteins (i.e., foods low in leucine). Fortunately, both groups can still overcome anabolic resistance by fortifying meals with about 3 grams of leucine.[18,19] All in all, these nutritional interventions to compensate for anabolic resistance are consistent with evidence-based recommendations that all adults should increase their consumption of high-quality protein for optimal muscle health (see Chapter 5).

Exercise, particularly resistance training, expressly functions by increasing the sensitivity of muscle to anabolic stimuli (e.g., leucine), thereby targeting the fundamental defect in aging muscle: an insensitivity to anabolic triggers. Even a single bout of resistance exercise followed by a leucine-rich essential amino acid recovery drink has been demonstrated to reverse age-related anabolic resistance.[1] For this reason, resistance exercise performed *prior* to consuming high-quality protein should be given high priority as being the most effective strategy to reverse anabolic resistance.[16]

In older adults, resistance exercise performed three times per week can build muscle, increase strength, and improve physical ability. Performing the same number of repetitions per set, older adults achieved greater gains in muscle strength and mass with high-intensity resistance exercise (heavy weights; 80% of maximum effort) compared with low-intensity resistance exercise (lighter weights; 40% of maximum effort). However, performing a higher number of repetitions at the lower intensity may result in equivalent gains in strength and mass *provided that the exercise is performed to muscle failure (fatigue).* Low-intensity exercise is particularly advantageous for older adults who are unable to lift heavy weights due to physical disabilities such as osteoarthritis.[20] See Chapter 7 for much more on exercise.

PART III

How to Preserve and Strengthen Your Muscle Mass

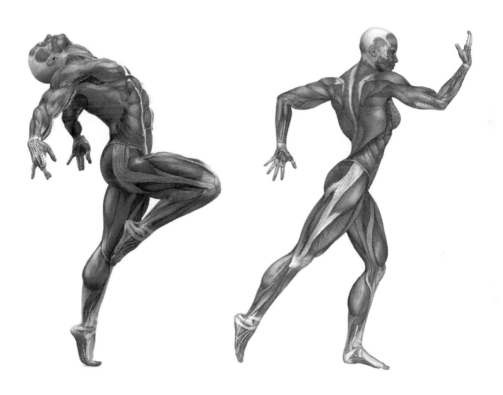

Chapter 7

Intense Exercise

The human body was designed to *move*. We evolved and adapted to the physically active lifestyle of our hunter-gatherer ancestors. The Hadza (present-day hunter-gatherers in northern Tanzania) are more physically active in a day than Americans are in an average week! Hunter-gatherers had to work hard and travel extensively to find food and survive. These behaviors were hardwired into our human genome to the extent that we need to stay physically active to be healthy.[1] *Exercise is mandatory, not optional—it is the* **sin qua non** *of muscle maintenance.*

Resistance training (RT) is the predominant type of exercise for developing and maintaining optimal muscle mass and strength. That said, while RT is clearly the superstar when it comes to muscle health, high-intensity interval training (HIIT) is a rising star. HIIT is primarily thought of as an alternative to continuous aerobic exercise for improving cardiorespiratory fitness, but new research suggests that this trendy and demanding workout also has the potential to increase muscle power, strength, and size.[2,3] A hallmark of both RT and HIIT is vigorous and exhausting effort. It is precisely this *intense effort* that makes these exercise strategies truly exceptional. Exercise is a powerful stimulus that causes the body to make physiological adaptations that improve health and fitness. However, these exercise adaptations are heavily influenced by exercise intensity. The higher-intensity exercise experience characteristic of HIIT and RT is associated with more robust adaptations; conversely, a lower-intensity exercise experience may not be sufficient to induce training adaptations in a substantial number of people.[4]

Beyond their muscle health benefits, regular participation in RT and HIIT can improve overall physical and mental health and reduce the risk of several chronic diseases, including cardiovascular disease, cancer, type 2 diabetes, osteoporosis, sarcopenia, and neurodegenerative diseases.[5,6] In a study of the effects of diverse types of exercise on gene expression, HIIT increased the expression of the largest number of health-enhancing genes (including genes regulating muscle growth), particularly in older adults. Several genes that decreased with age were reversed by HIIT, suggesting that intense exercise improves longevity.[4] Not to be outdone, 6 months of resistance training in healthy older adults produced a 50% increase in strength and caused the expression of 179 muscle genes associated with both age and exercise to markedly revert back to their "young" gene expression.[7] While light and moderate exercise certainly benefit many aspects of health, only vigorous exercise predicts longevity.[8]

When you perform intense exercise, your oxygen levels drop (hypoxia) to the point of losing your breath. We call that "getting winded." This low-energy state induces a hypoxic response that robustly triggers the activation of longevity regulators such as the sirtuins, a family of enzymes that have been shown to extend lifespan in yeast and mice. Sirtuins mediate the health benefits of exercise, including reduced oxidative stress and inflammation, creation of new muscle mitochondria and enhanced mitochondrial function, and improved DNA repair capability.[9,10] Experiments in mice suggest that sirtuins play a key role in the exercise-induced formation of new blood vessels (angiogenesis) that deliver essential oxygen and nutrients to muscles and other organs and tissues. Aging, however, causes the smallest blood vessels (capillaries) of the vasculature to shrivel and die off, resulting in reduced blood flow. This diminished blood flow from the loss of capillaries contributes to sarcopenia and other age-related diseases. Boosting sirtuin levels through intense exercise may be an effective anti-aging strategy to stimulate blood vessel growth and prevent muscle atrophy.[11]

Interestingly, exercise-induced lactate (from lactic acid) was shown in a mouse study to cross the blood-brain barrier and stimulate the production of nerve growth factor and the myokine BDNF (see Chapter 2) via the activation of a sirtuin gene called SIRT1. BDNF in turn mediates the benefits of exercise on brain health through improved learning and memory and reduced symptoms of depression.[12] *Notably, circulating lactate levels increase with exercise intensity.*

When all is said and done, pairing RT with HIIT provides the ultimate exercise duo in terms of boosting muscle health and general health as well as longevity.

Resistance Training

Resistance Training vs. Strength Training

While resistance training is also called "strength training," they are not exactly one and the same. "Resistance training" is a broad term comprising a variety of exercise subtypes that include strength training as well as power training, hypertrophy training, and muscular endurance training.

Now that you know how important resistance training is, let's talk more about it. RT is a conditioning strategy that involves working against some type of external resistance (load) in a progressive manner. The resistive load can be free weights (dumbbells and barbells), weight machines, elastic bands, medicine balls, your own body weight, or anything that causes muscle contraction. Since the demand or "overload" placed on the muscles is more intense than what they're accustomed to, damage occurs in the form of the microtearing of muscle fibers. However, after the initial muscle damage, growth mechanisms are triggered to repair the damage. This results in a greater increase in muscle protein synthesis (MPS) and stronger muscle fibers to manage the extra demand when the exercise is performed again. A progressive increase in overload (weight) may then induce the neuromuscular system to adapt by promoting muscle hypertrophy (growth).[13,14] Importantly, an adequate intake of high-quality protein—which also stimulates MPS—is essential for MPS to exceed muscle protein breakdown and result in a net gain in the production of muscle protein. Over time, the synergistic effects of consuming dietary protein *and* engaging in RT cause cumulative increases in MPS that ultimately lead to increases in muscle fiber size.[15,16]

When practiced consistently, RT that's progressively challenging produces multiple health benefits. This should be included in exercise programs for people of all ages! Beyond its long-recognized role in improving overall muscular fitness and athletic performance, RT can improve bone density, body composition, metabolic rate, insulin sensitivity, blood pressure, blood lipids, low back pain, arthritic discomfort, depression, anxiety, cognitive ability, and self-esteem. Accordingly, RT can play a major role in the prevention of metabolic diseases (e.g., cardiovascular disease, type 2 diabetes, colon cancer, metabolic syndrome) as well as osteoporosis, osteoarthritis, sarcopenia, and neurodegenerative disorders. Furthermore, both observational and interventional studies have demonstrated that RT can reduce the risk of dying from all causes.[17-19]

The 2018 Physical Activity Guidelines for Americans (issued by the U.S. Department of Health and Human Services), in accord with an American College of Sports Medicine (ACSM) position stand, include recommendations for resistance exercise. Adults of all ages should incorporate muscle-strengthening activities into their routine exercise regimen. These resistance exercises should target all of the major muscle groups—legs, hips, back, chest, abdomen, shoulders, and arms—and should be performed two or three nonconsecutive days per week to achieve optimal enhancement of muscle function and size. This training interval is based on research indicating that a rest period of 48 to 72 hours is necessary between sessions to allow molecular-level adaptations to stimulate the repair and growth of muscle tissue.[20,21] However, even a single exercise session per week has been shown to be sufficient in order for these adaptations to increase muscle size (see "Why Exercise Intensity is Critical").[22] In any case, the appropriate length of rest time between training sessions is highly dependent on the workout intensity and the related muscle damage.

In each workout session, individuals can train their entire body, or individuals can train different muscle groups in a "split-body" manner, such as alternating upper-body workouts with lower-body workouts. A "dose" of 1 set of 8 – 12 repetitions per muscle group can effectively increase muscle strength and size and may be especially appropriate for those who are new to resistance training. However, for most people, 2 – 4 sets per muscle group have been shown to be superior for muscle enhancement.[19,20] According to current evidence, a rest interval of 2 – 5 minutes between sets is required to achieve maximum muscular strength gains in resistance-trained individuals. In untrained individuals, however, short to moderate rest intervals (1 – 2 minutes) appear to be adequate for maximizing gains in muscular strength.[23]

Compound or multi-joint exercises engage more muscles with fewer exercises. Individuals can use five simple compound exercises that hit all of the major muscle groups as a solid foundation for their resistance training program (see Appendix). These core exercises are: the chest press, the seated row, the lat pulldown, the overhead press machine, and the leg press. The free-weight equivalents to these machine exercises include the barbell row, the overhead barbell/dumbbell press, the dead lift, the bench press, and the squat.

Proper exercise technique is essential! Resistance exercises should be performed in a measured and controlled manner to minimize momentum and should utilize a full range of motion of the joint. Attention should also be given to proper breathing, i.e., exhaling as the muscle shortens to raise the weight (concentric contraction) and inhaling when the muscle lengthens to lower the weight (eccentric contraction).[20] Another critical aspect of successful resistance training is muscle awareness and muscle control. Practice mindfulness—your mind-body connection—by first knowing which muscles or muscle groups you are working with each exercise

Muscle Quality

The quality of your muscle is just as critical as your muscle mass and strength. Defined as the amount of strength and/or power per unit of muscle mass, muscle quality in adults declines progressively with aging, contributing to deterioration in muscle function and mobility. In fact, decreases in muscle quality may even precede age-related losses of muscle mass.

One good predictor of poor muscle quality is insulin resistance in muscle. Fat infiltration within muscle tissue is one of the most important contributors to both poor muscle quality and insulin resistance within muscle. But the good news is that exercise—particularly resistance exercise—effectively increases muscle quality in both the young and the old, in part because exercise revives the capacity of muscle to burn *fat* in muscle mitochondria. As muscles are conditioned through resistance exercise, their quality improves and they become more insulin-sensitive, thus reversing insulin resistance and lowering the risk of chronic diseases. Once again, it's all about the muscle!

and then focusing solely on those muscles. For example, when performing the seated row (which primarily targets the back), concentrate on pulling with your back muscles and really *feel* those back muscles contracting. (See the Appendix for more information.) Since this is a compound exercise, other muscles such as your arm muscles will be secondarily engaged.

Exercises should be performed to muscular failure, which is the point at which another repetition is not possible. Reaching muscular failure (fatigue) triggers maximum muscle fiber activation, and this is fundamental for stimulating a substantial increase in muscle protein synthesis. High-intensity exercise performed to fatigue with full muscle fiber recruitment may be the key factor that underlies the muscle-building effects of resistance training.[24]

Why High-Intensity Exercise Is Critical

In resistance training, intensity is traditionally based on the load (weight) lifted as a percentage of a person's 1 RM, or "one repetition maximum." 1 RM is the maximum amount of weight that an individual can lift for only one repetition through a full range of motion. For example, the ACSM recommends RT intensities of about 70% – 80% of 1 RM for 8 – 12 repetitions to promote maximal muscle growth.[24] The load or intensity used in RT is only one of numerous other training variables for RT. These training variables include the choice of exercise, the order of exercise, an individual's training status, the time spent under tension, the number of sets/repetitions, an individual's speed of movement, and the duration of rest intervals between sets and exercises. This extreme variability allows individuals to pursue an endless number of different training sessions. Nevertheless, these different complex combinations of RT variables result in similar benefits for muscle and overall health.

Ultimately, it appears that one common and critical variable shared by these diverse RT protocols underlies their muscle-enhancing effects: *high intensity of effort*. In this context, exercise intensity is measured as the percentage or degree of *effort* rather than being conventionally defined as a percentage of 1 RM, along with the mindset that lifting heavy weights and not light weights is required to produce positive results.[25]

High Intensity of Effort

According to the traditional weightlifting paradigm of RT, an external load is the *exclusive* stimulus for building muscle bulk and strength. Under this model, heavier resistance (weight) is purported to be necessary to increase muscle protein synthesis and muscle mass during recovery. However, new research has demonstrated that when it comes to achieving increases in muscle size, training with lighter resistance is just as effective as training with heavier resistance *if the exercise is preformed to fatigue*.[24-26] Performing RT to momentary muscle fatigue—whether using heavy or light resistance or even with shorter or longer durations of repetitions—is the primary mediator of muscle growth. In other words, as long as muscle fatigue is achieved, heavier resistance (along with juggling countless other RT variables) is not necessary.[25]

Consistent with the focus on "training to fatigue," a newer and simpler paradigm has been proposed for RT, one that is based on an individual's own *effort* rather than an individual attempting to lift progressively heavier weights. This effort-based approach involves training with light to moderate weights to the point of muscle failure (fatigue) while maintaining excellent form. Even though heavy resistance is not utilized, putting forth a hard and challenging effort (which is internal to each individual) is still needed to target and reach the ultimate goal of muscle fatigue. In practice, individuals using RT and focusing on high-intensity effort can do a minimum of 1 set per exercise when said exercise utilizes core multi-joint exercises that target multiple muscle groups (see Appendix). Individuals employing this uncomplicated and time-efficient training model may see the same gains in muscle strength and growth that individuals who pursue the more intricate, time-consuming "heavy weight" model of resistance training see.[25,27]

According to evidence-based recommendations, individuals can achieve increases in muscle mass and strength by performing resistance training consistently and with a high intensity of effort, i.e., effort that is sufficient to reach muscle fatigue at the end of the set. These RT-induced muscle enhancements are not differentially impacted by sex or the multiple RT-related variables, although additional volume (repetitions x sets) may slightly improve muscle growth.[22] Note that sports-related performance such as power lifting may require heavier, near-maximal loads of greater than 85% 1 RM in order to maximize muscle strength. This is due to the specificity of training related to that sport.

Amazingly, even doing RT for 3 seconds per day—for example, a single bicep curl—for 5 days per week over a period of 4 weeks has been shown to increase muscle strength, again *provided that the training is performed at maximal effort!*[28]

So how exactly does muscle fatigue trigger muscles to increase in size and become stronger?

Fast-Twitch Muscle Fibers

At the cellular level, increases in muscle mass resulting from resistance training manifest as enlargement of muscle cells, a.k.a.

muscle fibers. Most people have an even mix of the two major types of muscle fiber in most of their muscles: slow-twitch (type I) and fast-twitch (type II). Slow-twitch fibers are ideally suited for low-intensity endurance (aerobic) exercise since they're packed with blood vessels, mitochondria, and oxygen-binding myoglobin; they are slow to fatigue and recover quickly. In contrast, fast-twitch fibers have more power and are better suited for anaerobic activities such as short, explosive bursts of strength (weightlifting) or speed (sprinting); however, they fatigue quickly and recover slowly.[27] Some elite distance runners and swimmers inherently have an exceptionally high percentage of slow-twitch fibers, whereas world-class sprinters may be naturally gifted with a larger proportion of fast-twitch fibers.[29]

Higher intensities of RT call into play (recruit) a greater number of muscle fibers to stimulate a strong MPS response and ultimately muscle growth. Both type I and type II fibers are engaged in resistance exercise. Since they require a small amount of energy, only the slow-twitch, low-threshold fibers are initially recruited in an attempt to move a resistance, namely to lift a weight. However, because slow-twitch fibers generate comparatively low levels of force, they're not capable of getting the job done, which in this case would be completing a lift. As the force increases, the more powerful fast-twitch, high-threshold fibers kick in to finish the job.[24,27]

Following high-intensity RT, type II fast-twitch muscle fibers have approximately 50% greater potential for gains in size compared with slow-twitch fibers.[30] Thus, type II fibers are the primary targets of RT regimens designed for promoting muscle growth. Resistance training with heavy-load resistance (greater than 60% of maximal strength) is known to activate and stimulate muscle growth in type II muscle fibers. Nevertheless, consistent with the effort-based model of RT, studies suggest that activation and subsequent size increase of type II fibers is implicit when RT is carried through to fatigue, independent of how much an individual lifts or what the repetition duration is. Furthermore, type I muscle fibers are activated just as much as type II fibers are.[26] In other words, when an individual performs RT to fatigue, their full spectrum of muscle fibers will be engaged.

Type II muscle fibers are more prone to atrophy than type I fibers are. Atrophy of type II muscle fibers accounts for the majority of muscle mass loss associated with aging and is a major hallmark of sarcopenia. The relative distribution of muscle fiber types shifts to the slower type I fibers with advancing age. With a smaller contribution made by high-powered type II fibers, the muscle strength of older adults is diminished, potentially leading to frailty, poor balance, and increased risk of falls and fractures.[31] Elderly females with hip fractures resulting from falls show extensive type II muscle fiber atrophy compared with healthy young or healthy elderly controls.[32]

Type II muscle fibers generate a lot of force to enable rapid, strong movements. Seeing as these fibers have a high threshold that can only be triggered by high-intensity exercise, it should come as no surprise that type II fibers shrink during aging. Among older adults who *do* work out regularly, few include high-intensity exercises in their routines. Thus, the lack of intense exercise in older age groups coupled with a lower intake of high-quality dietary protein (see Chapter 8) can contribute to age-related atrophy of the all-important type II muscle fibers.

Resistance training can counter muscle atrophy even when initiated later in life. In a study in older men ranging in age from 60 – 72 years, a 12-week strength-training program at 80% of maximum effort resulted in marked gains in muscle strength that was comparable to the strength gains observed in young men with an average age of 28 years. The older men also saw size increases in both their type I and their type II muscle fibers.[33] And even nonagenarians can get stronger! After following a similar high-intensity weight-training regimen for 8 weeks, frail nursing home residents up to age 96 achieved gains in muscle size and functional mobility. In particular, their strength improved by a dramatic 175%.[34]

Glycogen: More Than a Muscle Fuel

Glycogen is a large molecule made up of individual glucose units linked in a chain. It serves as the storage form of carbohydrate in muscle as well as in the liver. Muscle is the largest depository for glycogen, with type II fast-twitch muscle fibers having significantly higher concentrations of glycogen than type I slow-twitch fibers do.[35] While fat is the main fuel for muscles at rest and during light exercises such as slow walking, muscle glycogen comes increasingly into play as a fuel for moderately intense exercise, contributing just as much as fat does. As exercise reaches a high level of intensity, glycogen predominates, until eventually it is used exclusively.[36] Thus, high-intensity anaerobic exercise such as resistance training or sprinting—which primarily fires the glycogen-rich fast-twitch fibers—correspondingly causes considerable and rapid depletion of muscle glycogen stores, whereas low-intensity activity such as jogging uses glycogen more conservatively. In fact, muscle glycogen depletion associated with intense, all-out exercise can occur at a rate up to 40 times greater than the rate of glycogen breakdown related to low-intensity exercise (see graph below).[37]

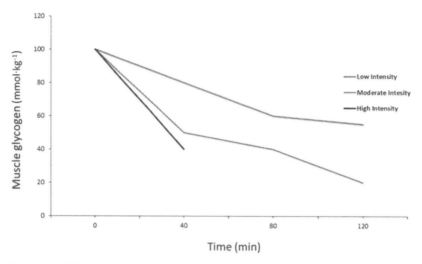

Reprinted with permission from Greene J., Louis J., Korostynska O., Mason A. State-of-the-Art Methods for Skeletal Muscle Glycogen Analysis in Athletes-The Need for Novel Non-Invasive Techniques. Biosensors. 2017;7:11.

In the liver, glycogen is converted to glucose and released into the blood to help maintain normal blood glucose levels and fuel other tissues. However, due to a lack of a specific enzyme, muscle cannot release glucose into the bloodstream; rather, muscle glycogen is metabolized on the spot for instant energy and is used only by muscle. Tapping muscle glycogen to fuel high-intensity exercise generates an enormous amount of energy to power fast-twitch muscle fibers. Muscle glycogen breakdown is stimulated by the stress hormone adrenaline, which is secreted *only* in muscles predominantly made up of fast-twitch fibers. One molecule of adrenaline is amplified during the flow of a cascade of reactions that ultimately results in the rapid mobilization of glycogen for immediate energy needs. *Importantly, muscle glycogen depletion has been shown to correlate significantly with muscle protein synthesis and muscle growth.*[26,38]

An increasingly popular training method used by endurance athletes involves *training* with low carbohydrate availability—that is, low glycogen stores—but *competing* with high glycogen stores. An endurance athlete's typical schedule consists of an evening workout followed by carbohydrate restriction overnight and then another training session the next morning. In accordance with this "train-low, compete-high" model, training adaptations induced by exercising in a glycogen-depleted state are enhanced compared to the same training adaptations associated with normal (or elevated) glycogen stores. These training adaptations include an increased capacity of muscle fibers to oxidize (burn) fat for fuel and thus potentially improve exercise performance.[35]

At the molecular level, training with low carbohydrate availability (or "training-low") enhances the expression of genes related to mitochondrial biogenesis, i.e., the generation of new mitochondria. With greater numbers of energy-producing mitochondria in muscle cells, each individual mitochondrion is able to share the "workload" and thus becomes more energy-efficient. To compensate for the lack of glycogen, the expanded mitochondrial content in muscle cells effectively adapts its energy-producing machinery to the burning of fat as a fuel.[39] In a study of well-trained cyclists, training with low muscle glycogen was shown to increase the metabolism of muscle-derived triglycerides (fats).[40] This major exercise adaptation may enable individuals to compete at higher intensities for longer durations.

The effects of improved mitochondrial function and other adaptations linked to training-low extend beyond athletic performance. As we age, mitochondria become functionally impaired. In turn, the buildup of inefficient mitochondria accelerates aging and underlies the development of age-related disorders. By recharging mitochondria, training-low slows aging and benefits overall health, including muscle health. Indeed, sarcopenia is associated with the defective turnover of mitochondria.[41]

In addition to driving the formation of new mitochondria, exercise (particularly intense exercise) also activates mitophagy, a "housekeeping" mechanism whereby damaged mitochondria are targeted for destruction and elimination. (Mitophagy is a form of *selective* autophagy). Thus, by restoring balance to the mitochondrial pool, exercise helps protect against muscle atrophy.[41] Exercising with low glycogen stores magnifies these adaptations.

Another notable adaptation associated with glycogen-depleting exercise is increased insulin sensitivity. It is well established that exercise conditions muscles to be more responsive to insulin. While this occurs immediately after a single bout of exercise and for up to 72 hours, continued exercise on a regular basis leads to sustained improvement in insulin sensitivity. Increased insulin sensitivity and the accompanying improvement in **blood sugar control** contribute to the benefits of exercise in preventing and treating type 2 diabetes.[38] In addition, improved insulin sensitivity reinforces the enhanced fat-burning capacity of muscle that's associated with training with low glycogen. Specifically, lower circulating levels of insulin resulting from increased insulin sensitivity enable greater oxidation (burning) of fat during exercise.[37] (On the flip side, high insulin levels caused by insulin resistance drive fat accumulation.)

The amount of muscle glycogen used up during exercise plays a central role in insulin action. Insulin's ability to move glucose into muscle post-exercise is positively correlated to the degree of glycogen depletion caused by the exercise. The more glycogen that's used up (as with intense exercise), the stronger the insulin signal becomes (greater sensitivity). The enhanced metabolic action of insulin to stimulate glucose entry into muscle drives replenishment or even "supercompensation" of the muscle glycogen deficit. Partial or full restoration of glycogen stores occurs even without *any* food intake during exercise recovery (i.e., carbs during recovery are not necessary to replete glycogen; see Chapter 5). The buildup of lactate (from lactic acid) that results from fatiguing exercise is a likely precursor for the synthesis of glycogen. From an evolutionary perspective, the insulin-mediated restoration of depleted muscle glycogen may have been a high-priority survival adaptation that provided our hunter-gatherer ancestors with emergency energy for "fight-or-flight" situations like running from predators.[42]

So is it better to keep our muscle glycogen tanks "topped up," so to speak?

Oddly enough, no. While maintaining full glycogen stores was likely a critical adaptation for our ancient ancestors, it can have adverse consequences in our modern world of food abundance and inactivity. When muscle glycogen stores become full, excess blood glucose—generally caused by consuming too many carbs— is diverted to synthesize fat in the liver. This can lead to a rise in levels of LDL cholesterol and triglycerides as well as a reduction in beneficial HDL levels. The conversion of excess glucose to fat can also cause a buildup of fat within muscle, which can promote the subsequent development of muscle insulin resistance.[38,43] Recall that insulin resistance contributes to sarcopenia and is associated with several metabolic disorders such as type 2 diabetes, cardiovascular disease, and cancer.

Paradoxically, too much muscle glycogen may even *decrease* exercise endurance! In an experimental mouse study, mice that were genetically manipulated to have an overaccumulation of muscle glycogen unexpectedly became exhausted faster than control mice when performing strenuous exercise. The mutant mice also exhibited a comparatively lower resting metabolic rate (RMR), suggesting that the capacity of these mice to burn glucose or fat for energy was lower at rest. Researchers determined that the slow-twitch endurance muscle fibers from the soleus muscle of the mutant mice switched their metabolism to the metabolism of fast-twitch fibers. The normally slow-to-fatigue soleus fibers displayed impaired aerobic metabolism and—again like fast-twitch fibers—less resistance to fatigue and decreased muscle endurance.[44]

In Summary

Let's now sum up and tie together this somewhat complex discussion of the special muscle benefits of high-intensity exercise. Consistently performing resistance exercise with a high enough degree of effort to cause *muscle fatigue* maximizes muscle mass and strength. Intense exercise primarily recruits the fast-twitch muscle fibers, which have greater potential for muscle growth than slow-twitch fibers do. Stronger and bulkier fast-twitch fibers, in turn, improve an individual's ability to perform resistance exercise. These fast-twitch fibers are also loaded with glycogen, which provides as much as 80% of the energy used during resistance training.

The depletion of muscle glycogen stores to fuel muscle is greatly accelerated during high-intensity exercise (compared with low-intensity exercise). This considerable drainage of muscle glycogen, amplified by adrenaline, prompts a proportionate boost in glycogen synthesis to replenish its stores. Muscle glycogen depletion is also related to the activation of proteins that signal muscle protein synthesis and to the subsequent growth of fast-twitch muscle fibers.

Not surprisingly, however, exercise performance is impaired when glycogen stores are reduced to a certain degree. Having a high amount of muscle glycogen prior to athletic competitions is desirable. Intense training maximizes the capacity of muscle to store glycogen to support and enhance exercise performance.

Nevertheless, the strategy of deliberately exercising noncompetitively with low glycogen stores can be used periodically to enhance the training adaptations associated with exercising with normal glycogen levels. These enhanced adaptations include an improved fat-burning capacity of muscle during exercise and an increased whole-body insulin sensitivity, both of which reinforce each other.

Ultimately, keeping your muscle glycogen stores *below* the full level is linked to good metabolic health. *Intermittent* emptying of muscle glycogen stores through intense exercise (along with a low carb intake) is the optimal way to ensure that muscle glycogen stores remain incompletely full. The upshot is that more robust exercise adaptations lead to increased insulin sensitivity and the prevention of insulin resistance and all of its associated disorders. In one study, insulin sensitivity was improved by 85% following high-intensity exercise versus just 51% following moderate-intensity exercise.[45]

On the other hand, low-intensity, steady-state exercises such as running, jogging, or swimming do not engage glycogen-rich fast-twitch muscle fibers and thereby do not typically exhaust muscle glycogen content to a significant extent. Without available storage space, excess blood glucose is converted to fat and muscle cells begin to develop insulin resistance. (Again, excess blood glucose is caused by consuming too many carbs.)

Strengthening the Heart Muscle, Too: The Compelling Aerobic Benefits of Resistance Exercise

It's been well established that resistance training is the go-to exercise for increasing the strength and mass of our skeletal muscles, whereas endurance (aerobic) exercise is the preferred training method for targeting and strengthening the heart muscle. However, you may be surprised to find out that your weightlifting session will not only improve your muscular strength but your cardio health as well! Research has shown that resistance training induces a marked improvement in cardiovascular fitness.[46]

Cardiovascular Risk

Multiple studies have shown that resistance exercise has equal or greater effects than aerobic activities when it comes to reducing cardiovascular risk factors in both young and older adults. Compared with aerobic exercise, resistance training has been shown to have a stronger association with improvements in hypertension, blood lipid profiles, and the development of diabetes.[47] Indirectly, the cardioprotective effects of resistance exercise are attributed to its profound enhancement of skeletal muscle health. As detailed in Chapter 2, muscle plays an essential role in metabolic health, including cardiovascular health. For example, muscle is the primary driver of resting metabolic rate (RMR) and is a major contributor to insulin sensitivity and *blood sugar control*. These factors—as well as metabolic flexibility and appropriate myokine secretion—are associated with greater fat burning and lower inflammation, both of which in turn reduce cardiovascular risk.

But how exactly does RT improve aerobic fitness, i.e., the ability of the heart and lungs to deliver oxygen to working muscles?

Aerobic Fitness

Before we answer this question, let us once again more accurately define the intensity of RT as the point of maximal *effort* (rather than *load*) when momentary muscular failure (fatigue) is reached. A strong case can be made that improvements in cardiovascular fitness are primarily dependent on the *intensity* of the exercise and are independent of the *type* of exercise. Accordingly, in studies of RT performed to muscle failure, both young and older adults experienced substantial improvements in VO2 max, which is the maximal amount of oxygen that the body can transport and utilize during intense exercise. VO2 max is the most valid marker for cardiorespiratory fitness. Another cardiovascular adaptation induced by pursuing RT to the point of muscle failure is the development and proliferation of a network of capillaries within muscles. This improves cardiovascular fitness by significantly increasing blood flow and oxygen supply to muscles.[46]

The Metabolic Link

The RT-induced enhancements in VO2 max and blood flow are easy to appreciate. On the other hand, the *metabolic* link between anaerobic exercise and aerobic exercise is not widely recognized…yet it is fascinating. Anaerobic metabolism occurs without utilizing oxygen; it is traditionally associated with short bursts of intense activity such as what we experience during resistance training, jumping, and sprinting. Aerobic metabolism, in contrast, requires oxygen to generate energy and is generally characteristic of endurance activities such as running, swimming, and bicycling. However, these two energy systems overlap and usually work together, though one system carries more weight and thereby defines the activity (i.e., the activity is referred to as being an "aerobic" or "anaerobic" one). The *intensity* of the exercise is the primary factor that determines which system dominates.[46]

Here's where things get really interesting. All aerobic exercise begins with a contribution from anaerobic metabolism via glycolysis. Anaerobic glycolysis is the metabolic pathway that breaks down glucose (in the absence of oxygen) to a compound called pyruvate, releasing energy in the process. The pyruvate formed by this anaerobic process is then used to fuel the slower but much more energy-efficient aerobic (utilizing oxygen) processes that take place in the mitochondria, the cell's power plants. (This sequence of chemical reactions is called the Krebs cycle.) As explained by Dr. Doug McGuff, author of the best-selling book *Body by Science*, "The only way to get your cardiovascular system to work harder is by performing mechanical work with muscle." The greater the intensity of the exercise (mechanical work), the higher the rate of pyruvate entry into the mitochondria to power the aerobic cycle. This being the case, unlike high-intensity training, low-intensity steady-state cardio workouts do not *maximally* stimulate aerobic metabolism.[27]

Since glycolysis produces energy (and pyruvate) 100 times faster than aerobic energy production in the mitochondria does, eventually the pyruvate production will exceed the capacity of the mitochondria to process it. The surplus of unused pyruvate is converted to lactate (lactic acid). Contrary to popular belief, lactate is greatly beneficial! It is *not* harmful to muscle function and metabolism during intense exercise. Most of the lactate is subsequently converted back to pyruvate and processed aerobically in muscle mitochondria.[36] Some lactate is released into the bloodstream to be used to fuel other organs and tissues such as the heart and brain.[48] The more physically active you are, the greater capacity you'll have to utilize lactate as a fuel. That's because exercise appears to increase the number of specific transporters that facilitate entry of lactate into cells.

Beyond its role as a fuel, lactate appears to play an important role as a signaling molecule that mediates many exercise-induced adaptations, including muscle growth.[49] Lactate administered to mice has been shown to induce muscle growth and regeneration by stimulating the activation of muscle satellite (stem) cells and their maturation into muscle fibers.[52] Lactate has also been shown to activate protein synthesis factors such as mTOR in skeletal muscle of rats.[50]

The effects of lactate on muscle health are also linked to the release of myokines from muscle cells (see Chapter 2). Lactate increases the secretion of BDNF (brain-derived neurotrophic factor)[51] but suppresses myostatin.[52] While BDNF contributes to the regeneration of exercise-induced muscle damage, myostatin promotes muscle breakdown and is associated with muscle atrophy. Interestingly, consuming antioxidants has been shown to reverse the effects induced by lactate, suggesting that the benefits of lactate are driven by free radicals (ROS).[49]

Essentially, the linkage between anaerobic and aerobic training is made clear by the metabolism of both pyruvate and lactate during exercise: the byproducts of one energy system (anaerobic) are used to fuel the other system (aerobic).[48] This enhancement of aerobic fitness induced by RT occurs during recovery, when the "afterburn" kicks in. The increased energy expenditure from the afterburn effect—referred to as the "excess post-exercise oxygen consumption" or EPOC—is used to restore the body back to a pre-exercise state and allows for the aerobic processing (oxidation) of lactate. A key aspect of EPOC is that it increases exponentially as the intensity of exercise increases.[53] A systematic review of studies concluded that high-intensity interval training results in greater EPOC than moderate-intensity continuous aerobic exercise does.[54] Since this increased stimulation of the aerobic system via EPOC is intensity-driven and *not* dependent on the type of exercise, it's reasonable to expect that pursuing RT to muscle failure will result in comparable aerobic benefits. And in fact, EPOC has been reported to last up to 72 hours after RT.[55]

The Muscle Fiber Link

Another notable adaptation to resistance exercise that increases muscle aerobic capacity is a change in muscle fiber behavior.

A particular subset of fast-twitch fibers is capable of both anaerobic and aerobic energy production. Known as "fast-oxidative-glycolytic" (FOG) fibers, these fibers contribute to the increased aerobic capacity that's induced by RT. Studies support a shift in muscle fiber activity from predominantly anaerobic toward FOG as a result of RT performed to failure.[46] Increases in muscle fiber size (muscle mass gains) resulting from RT have also been associated with increased muscle aerobic capacity.[56] Conversely, in a study of older adults, subjects with sarcopenia (muscle mass loss) were found to have lower measures of cardiorespiratory fitness (VO2 max) than subjects without sarcopenia.[57] These findings provide evidence that an increase/decrease in muscle mass necessitates a corresponding increase/decrease in the capacity of the cardiorespiratory system to "service" it with fuel and oxygen when muscles are contracting. Furthermore, the higher the *intensity* of contracting muscles is (e.g., via RT or HIIT), the harder the heart and lungs need to work and the greater the improvement in aerobic capacity will be.

The Molecular Link

Finally, without delving too far into molecular biology, it's especially interesting to learn how the underlying molecular mechanisms involved in RT support its ability to improve aerobic fitness. AMPK (AMP-activated protein kinase) and mTOR are two major signaling proteins with opposing actions. They're mutually exclusive, meaning that when one is activated, the other one is inhibited. Whereas AMPK is catabolic (obtaining energy from breaking down stored fat) and featured in endurance exercise, mTOR is anabolic (consuming energy to build proteins and grow) and is linked to RT. *During* intense exercise such as RT to failure, AMPK is activated (to regenerate energy) in response to low cellular energy resulting from the high rate of fuel usage from the intense effort. Concurrently, mTOR is inhibited to minimize energy consumption that would otherwise drive anabolic effects such as muscle growth. *After* resistance exercise, however, a delayed activation of mTOR occurs that promotes the expected increase in muscle growth and strength. At the same time, this activation shuts off the catabolic effects of AMPK. (As discussed in Chapter 5, high-quality animal protein such as whey should be consumed in a post-exercise recovery beverage or meal to maximize the anabolic effect.) In essence, at the molecular level, when associated with RT to failure, the initial and delayed activations of AMPK and mTOR respectively drive improvements in aerobic fitness as well as muscle growth and strength.[46]

High-Intensity Interval Training (HIIT)

HIIT has become a widely used, effective, and time-efficient alternative to traditional aerobic exercise. It involves short, intermittent bursts of vigorous exercise interspersed with recovery periods of rest or lower-intensity exercise. Typically, a high-intensity interval workout consists of intense effort for 5 seconds – 8 minutes performed at 80% – 90% of maximal heart rate (submaximal). These short bouts of exercise are separated by 1 – 3 minutes of recovery at low intensity or by complete rest. A single workout session of alternating exercise and recovery continues for 3 – 4 cycles (totaling 20 – 60 minutes) performed 2 – 3 times per week. Any exercise mode (e.g., cycling, walking, swimming) can be adapted for HIIT workouts. [58] A more demanding version of HIIT is sprint interval training (SIT) characterized by a 30-second "all-out" (supramaximal) effort followed by a longer recovery of 4 – 5 minutes. With warm-up and cool-down, 4 cycles of SIT can be completed in 25 minutes, of which only 2 minutes are intense. As SIT is extremely strenuous, it's more appropriate for athletes and physically fit individuals.[59]

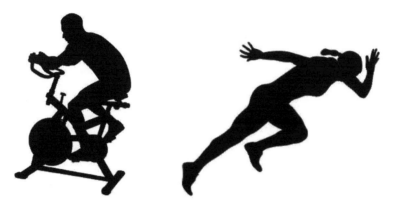

Super1973/shutterstock.com Copyright: spotpoint74

Better Than Conventional Cardio

Multiple studies have demonstrated that HIIT workouts are superior to moderate-intensity continuous exercise when it comes to improving aerobic fitness and reducing cardiovascular risk factors such as insulin resistance and inflammation.[60] In fact, in people with chronic diseases caused by poor lifestyle, HIIT was nearly *twice* as effective at increasing cardiorespiratory fitness than moderate-intensity steady-state cardio![61] What's more, HIIT is very time-efficient, which is particularly worth noting since "a lack of time" is one of the most frequent reasons that people give when asked why they avoid exercising.

HIIT Promotes Muscle Growth

If the impressive aerobic fitness benefits of HIIT alone weren't enough, evidence also suggests that this quick (albeit challenging) workout is a promising approach for building and maintaining muscle mass. That's because HIIT has been shown to stimulate cellular and molecular mechanisms that eventually lead to muscle growth. For example, HIIT and SIT can modulate the expression of specific genes and proteins associated with the regulation of muscle mass. Moreover, HIIT can activate muscle satellite (stem) cells and boost muscle protein synthesis (MPS).[62]

In one study, MPS in response to different types of exercise was determined in sedentary older men around 67 years old. While resistance training (RT) resulted in the greatest increase in MPS, HIIT was also found to induce significant increases in MPS, though not to the same extent. No increase in MPS was observed after conventional aerobic exercise.[2] Similar increases in MPS were observed in young adults with an average age of 23 years after 3 weeks of SIT.[63]

As discussed previously, gains in muscle mass occur when MPS exceeds muscle protein breakdown over a prolonged period. In all likelihood, the enhanced MPS following weeks/months of repeated HIIT would lead to gains in muscle mass. Many studies have shown that short-term and prolonged HIIT across a range of age groups results in increases in lean/fat-free mass, which is a proxy for changes in muscle mass. However, many other studies did *not* find changes in lean/fat-free mass.[62] An important omission in most of the negative studies was the availability of dietary protein—the amount, type, and timing of protein consumption was *not* factored into the results. With this in mind, it's worth recalling that when coupled with repeated sessions of RT, protein consumption results in a buildup of muscle protein and increased muscle mass. HIIT resembles RT in that they both involve high-intensity muscle contractions that cause damage to muscle fibers, thus necessitating repair and subsequent protein synthesis. Both types of exercise also induce greater activation of type II muscle fibers, which have the highest potential for growth. High priority should be given to future studies examining the capacity for HIIT *paired with high-quality dietary protein* to promote muscle growth.[62]

Finally, recall that lactate stimulates the activation of muscle stem cells as well as mTOR-the master regulator of muscle protein synthesis. High-intensity exercise such as HIIT is one surefire way to make your lactate levels soar!

HIIT Enhances Muscle Strength and Power

HIIT also improves muscle strength and muscle power. Significant increases in knee extensor strength were observed in healthy young men (mean age 29 years) after 6 sessions of all-out HIIT performed on a cycle ergometer over a 2-week period. In contrast, no improvement in the strength of the knee extensors was observed in those participants who completed 6 sessions of continuous cycling for up to 2 hours at low to moderate intensity.[64]

Muscle power is the product of strength + speed, i.e., the ability to exert a force quickly. Examples of muscle power include explosive jumping, sprinting, throwing, and the snatch in weightlifting. Muscle power diminishes more abruptly than muscle strength during aging and is thus a stronger determinant of future falls, loss of autonomy in older adults, and even death.

A 5-week HIIT-based running plan enhanced athletic performance in a group of triathletes by improving muscle power. Greater muscle power was evidenced by faster sprinting and swimming times as well as improved jumping performance.[65] Older, nonathletic adults can also improve muscle power via HIIT, though with longer recovery periods. In a study of sedentary men between 57 and 67 years old, 6 weeks of HIIT performed every 5 days was shown to be both achievable and effective as an exercise regimen for significantly improving leg muscle power.[3]

Documented health benefits of high-intensity interval training

| Improves mood and decreases feelings of depression and anxiety |
| Lower risk of breast cancer |
| Lower risk of cardiovascular disease |
| Increases metabolic rate and lowers body fat mass |
| Reduction in incident osteoarthritis |

| Lower risk of metabolic sendrome |
| Helps relief from low back pain |
| Improves insulin sensitivity and lower risk of T2D |
| Lower risk of colon cancer |
| Reduction in falls for older people |

Reprinted from: Atakan MM, Li Y, Kosar SN, Turnagol HH, Yan X. Evidence-based effects of high-intensity interval training on exercise capacity and health: a review with historical perspective. Int J Environ Res Public Health. 2021;18(13):7201.

What About Steady-State Cardio?

As previously mentioned, aerobic exercise—otherwise known as "steady-state" or "continuous" cardio—is considered to be the exercise of choice for improving cardiorespiratory fitness. Resistance training, in contrast, primarily enhances muscle size and strength. However, RT clearly improves cardiorespiratory (aerobic) fitness as well. So does conventional aerobic training exert a similar crossover effect and induce muscle growth?

© Glasbergen/ glasbergen.com

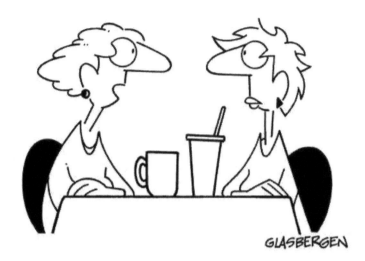

GLASBERGEN

"I do weights for muscle health, cardio for heart health and chocolate for mental health."

Studies have demonstrated that aerobic exercise training can in fact promote an increase in muscle size.[66,67] But in line with the main theme of this chapter, a *high intensity of effort* is likely to be essential to achieve muscle growth from endurance exercise. Specifically, this means training with 70% – 80% of maximal effort for a duration of 30 – 45 minutes with a frequency of 4 – 5 days per week.[66] This is not like going out for an easy run or jog! Rather, it is a *tempo* run that feels like a 6 – 8 on an Effort Scale of 1 – 10, with 1 being walking. This medium level of intensity is often described as "comfortably hard," i.e., talking should be limited to short sentences. The same intensity level applies to cycling and other modes of exercise as well. Exercising at 70% – 80% of one's maximum heart rate is also considered "lactate threshold training," whereby lactate is cleared as fast as it is produced such that blood levels of lactate remain constant. Training beyond the lactate threshold leads to short-term exhaustion.

Nevertheless, when it comes to promoting muscle growth, RT is significantly superior to conventional cardio. This is consistent with popular belief and not unexpected. A systematic review and meta-analysis of 21 studies concluded that aerobic exercise does not induce the same increase in knee extensor muscle size as RT does. Though sufficient data was only available for the knee extensor muscles, the superior muscle-building effects of RT likely extend to other muscle groups as well. One reason might be that the multiple exercises involved in RT enable greater activation of distinct muscle groups compared with cardio exercises such as running or cycling.[68]

An important difference between the two exercise modes that may also partly explain the superior muscle growth associated with RT involves the recruitment of muscle fibers. According to the same 21-study review, RT is more effective than cardio at increasing the size of both the fast-twitch type II muscle fibers and the slow-twitch type I fibers. During exercise, motor units (groups of identical-twitch muscle fibers innervated by a single nerve) are recruited sequentially according to size. The smaller slow-twitch motor units are fired first, followed by the larger fast-twitch units as intensity increases. Proper RT performed to muscular failure in a deliberate and controlled manner will sequentially tap into all available muscle fibers, ultimately engaging the higher-threshold fast-twitch fibers that have the greatest potential to increase in size. On the other hand, continuous submaximal cardio primarily stimulates the smaller lower-threshold motor units that are slow to fatigue and quick to recover. Thus, cardio exercise cycles through the smaller motor units repeatedly and in such a way that the fast-twitch fibers are not necessarily stimulated. Disuse of fast-twitch muscle fibers over time may lead to loss of muscle mass and reduced glycogen storage capacity, resulting in "topped-up" muscle glycogen stores. As a consequence, the risk of developing insulin resistance and related metabolic disorders may increase (especially when the diet is high carb).[27,68]

At the molecular level, aerobic and resistance training stimulate different types of muscle protein synthesis and differ in their ability to activate post-exercise signaling proteins that regulate muscle growth. In general, RT increases strength and muscle fiber size, which is associated with *myofibrillar* protein. By comparison, aerobic exercise increases endurance in part by boosting levels of energy-producing mitochondria in muscle, thus increasing muscle *mitochondrial* protein. (The latter is nonetheless a great health benefit!) Accordingly, in a study of young and healthy men, pursuing RT for 10 weeks increased myofibrillar but not muscle mitochondrial protein synthesis, whereas endurance training stimulated the synthesis of muscle mitochondrial but not myofibrillar protein.[69] Furthermore, while a key mTOR-dependent signaling pathway was activated by acute bouts of both exercise modes, it remained above resting levels at 4 hours *after RT only*. Recall that signaling by the mTOR protein is highly correlated with RT-induced gains in muscle size.

For superior overall muscle maintenance, the take-home message is to be sure to include resistance training in your exercise regimen. Do not limit yourself to just doing purely aerobic activities!

For much more on this topic, see the Appendix for one of the best books you will ever read on the importance of intense exercise: *Body by Science* by Doug McGuff and John Little.

For Maximal Benefits, Exercise When Fasting

According to Stephen Anton, PhD, a leading authority on intermittent fasting, exercising in the fasted state may boost muscle growth and endurance.[70] Exercise and fasting are mild stresses to the body—meaning that they mimic adversity—that activate adaptive stress responses to increase disease and stress resistance. They also improve physical and cognitive performance. This phenomenon is called "hormesis" (see Chapter 9).

Depletion of liver glycogen through fasting generates ketones, which help preserve muscle mass. Meanwhile, muscle glycogen depletion via exercise drives muscle protein synthesis and muscle growth. For good measure, when glycogen stores are exhausted, muscle becomes trained to burn fat more efficiently for energy. Both of these intermittent challenges increase the insulin sensitivity of muscle cells, and this in turn enhances muscle health. All in all, exercising while fasting results in a doubling-down effect— the improvements in muscle and overall health that result from pursuing both challenges concurrently are superior to the results obtained from pursuing those individual challenges alone.

Chapter 8

Up the Protein, Lower the Carbs

There was a sick man of Tobago,
Liv'd long on rice-gruel and sago;
But at last to his bliss,
The physician said this—
"To a roast leg of mutton you may go."

—John Marshall, c. 1821

It is implicit that the best diet for promoting optimal muscle health is also the most effective eating pattern for overall health maintenance, disease prevention, and longevity. As discussed in Chapters 4 and 5, a low-carbohydrate/higher-protein diet (35% – 40% carbohydrate; 30% – 35% protein) is more effective than a high-carbohydrate/lower-protein ratio (55% – 60% carbohydrate; 12% – 15% protein) for maintaining muscle mass and improving body composition. While our total daily protein intake is the most important factor, the quantity *and quality* of protein we need to consume to maximize our muscle health can be conveniently expressed by the concept of a meal-based threshold. Accordingly, a protein intake of 30 – 50 grams 3 times each day is optimal for supporting not only muscle health but other protein functions as well (e.g., blood sugar control, appetite regulation). To ensure high quality, the protein should contain the complete and balanced assortment of essential amino acids, including about 3 grams of leucine. This is more easily and effectively achieved by eating animal protein (which offers fewer calories and zero carbs) than the larger, more caloric amounts of carbohydrate-rich plant proteins that would be needed to provide the same dose of leucine.

Beyond muscle health, there's compelling evidence that diets lower in carbohydrate content improve cardiovascular risk factors (e.g., hypertension, high blood fats, and inflammation) and are safe and effective in the management of type 2 diabetes. A low-carbohydrate diet appears to also protect against cancer[1,2] as well as Alzheimer's disease and Parkinson's disease.[3]

Protein Is First and Foremost

The word "protein" originates from the Greek term *proteios*, meaning "the first rank."[4] When planning a meal, the first macronutrient to consider is protein. *Protein is the core of your meal.* Everything else (e.g., vegetables, fruits, fats) should be centered around your protein food(s). Indeed, we humans—along with numerous other animals—have an instinctive appetite for protein. We have feedback mechanisms that enable us to adjust our diet to maintain a relatively constant intake of protein. For example, when the percentage of protein in our diet is low, we'll overeat carbohydrates and fats in order to obtain more of the high-priority protein. This instinctive mechanism unfortunately favors weight gain and obesity. Conversely, when we eat a diet with a high percentage of protein (30% of our total calories), we're more satiated and we require less food to obtain sufficient protein. This creates an energy deficit and possible weight loss. The tendency to prioritize protein when regulating food intake is referred to as the "protein leverage hypothesis."[5,6]

An analysis of data from the CDC's National Health and Nutrition Examination Survey (NHANES) provides evidence to support the protein leverage hypothesis. During both the HANES I (1971 – 1975) and HANES 2005 – 2006 surveys, an increase in the percentage of calories from protein strongly and consistently correlated with a decrease in daily caloric intake in normal-weight, overweight, and obese adults.[7] As discussed in Chapter 4, this is consistent with studies reporting greater weight loss and muscle retention in people who eat diets with a high protein-to-carbohydrate ratio versus people who eat diets with the reverse ratio.

People eating diets considerably higher in protein than what people eat in modern-day Western countries (which are beset by an epidemic of obesity and diabetes) is not a foreign concept within human history and evolution. Over the last 700,000 years marked by various Ice Ages, early humans subsisted primarily by hunting and fishing, becoming increasingly carnivorous. Our hunter-gatherer ancestors evolved on a low-carbohydrate, high-protein carnivorous diet interspersed by periods of famine. Paleolithic humans thrived on an average protein intake of 37% of total calories,[8] dwarfing the current average protein consumption of 15% of dietary energy. Their estimated carbohydrate consumption primarily came from seasonal roots and berries and ranged from a paltry 10 grams per day up to 125 grams per day. Again, this is a far cry from today's average daily carb intake of 250 – 400 grams.[9]

Researchers have hypothesized that chronic consumption of a high-protein, low-carbohydrate diet may lead to decreased utilization of glucose by peripheral muscle tissue, thereby sparing glucose for preferential fueling of other tissues such as the brain. In other words, this muscle- and health-promoting diet may cause muscle insulin resistance. Confused? But there's actually a rational explanation for this seemingly counterintuitive statement. Insulin resistance induced by a high-protein, low-carb diet is not the *pathological* insulin resistance associated with chronic present-day diseases because the compensatory increased secretion of insulin to maintain normal blood glucose is not needed (due to eating few to no carbs). Rather, this *physiological* insulin resistance is our body's way of adapting to a low-carb diet by prioritizing vital glucose for the brain.[9] The brain uses fat-derived ketones for a large portion of its energy needs when dietary carbs are significantly reduced; nevertheless, it still requires some glucose.

According to the aptly named "carnivore connection" hypothesis, insulin resistance became a survival and reproductive advantage during the various Ice Ages when dietary carbohydrates were scarce. During pregnancy, insulin resistance enabled glucose to be diverted from skeletal muscles to the fetus and mammary gland, thereby increasing birth weight and the survival of the next generation. Fast-forward to modern times featuring easy and continuous access to highly refined, high-glycemic carbohydrates paired with inactivity, and you have an epidemic of pathological insulin resistance characterized by substantially elevated blood insulin levels. It is the *combination* of insulin resistance and high blood insulin (hyperinsulinemia) that predisposes people to obesity and associated metabolic diseases such as type 2 diabetes and cardiovascular disease.[10] Context is everything.

With respect to muscle health, higher protein consumption among older adults predicts muscle mass and strength and counters the development of sarcopenia. According to a systematic review and meta-analysis of randomized controlled trials in adults aged 50 and over who did resistance exercises, increased protein intake results in greater lean mass and strength when compared with control participants who consume lower amounts of protein.[11] This association between increased dietary protein and greater lean mass and muscle strength has also been observed in middle-aged adults, although interventional studies are needed to substantiate this finding.[12]

High-Quality Animal Protein Is Essential

Protein is the stuff we're all made of—it's the building blocks of life. But not all dietary proteins are created equal. Our muscles deserve the highest-quality protein possible to function optimally and maintain themselves! Animal proteins from meats, fish, eggs, and dairy are clearly superior to plant proteins, particularly with regard to muscle protein synthesis and maintenance of muscle mass. So why settle for low-quality plant protein?

Collagen Is Animal Protein

Collagen is our most abundant protein, making up about one-third of the body's total protein mass. Basically, collagen is the "glue" that holds us together. It's a structural protein found throughout the body, primarily in connective tissues such as cartilage, bones, tendons, ligaments, and skin. Collagen acts as a scaffold for bone cells onto which calcium is deposited. While we generally don't associate collagen with muscle, about 10% of skeletal muscles are comprised of collagen—it's critical for their structure and function.

Animal foods have comprised a large proportion of our human diet for millennia. A diet lacking in animal protein can result in nutritional deficiencies, leading to poor muscle growth and health. In a study of housebound elderly people, those who consumed less than 65% of their total protein from animal foods became deficient in at least one essential amino acid, resulting in protein malnutrition.[13] And high-quality animal protein is absolutely critical for growing children! An excellent example of this can be seen in data from China: between 1990 and 2010, the consumption of animal-sourced foods in China increased by 115%. During this 20-year period, the prevalence of growth stunting in children under 5 years of age decreased from 33% to 9.5%.[14]

Unfortunately, the public is generally unaware of the many important advantages that animal protein has over plant protein (see Chapter 5). This lack of knowledge is reflected in the fact that plant-based and vegan diets are rising sharply in popularity. People following these diets may often feel better initially, but that has nothing to do with the avoidance of animal foods, which is a practice that poses severe health risks in the long run. Rather, people most likely feel better because they're eliminating sugars and processed, high-glycemic junk foods while switching to a whole-food diet. No civilization in human history has lived on a diet that was 100% free of animal foods. Consider Okinawa, one of the world's "Blue Zones," a designation given to places where people live the longest. The people of Okinawa are celebrated for eating a plant-based diet, which is claimed to be the key to their longevity. However, Okinawans also regularly consume seafood along with small amounts of lean meats and dairy.[15]

Meanwhile, some current indigenous peoples have flourished almost exclusively on an animal food diet with little or virtually no plant food. These hunter-gatherers (e.g., the Masai and Hadza tribes of Africa and the Inuit of the Arctic regions) have low rates of chronic diseases such as heart disease and cancer.[16] Interestingly, while the Hadza consume generous amounts of honey—as well as baobab fruit, berries, and tubers—they rarely eat greens. The energy cost of foraging for greens was likely historically higher than the energy (calories) they provided.[17]

Many people today are reluctant to eat meat, dairy, and eggs… which is ironic seeing as these are the most nutritious foods on the planet for human consumption. Sadly, people are being continuously misled by negative and flawed observational studies sensationalized by the media, studies that incriminate animal protein and particularly meat as being unhealthy and disease-promoting. In a prime example, an observational study of 6,381 U.S. adults aged 50 and above concluded that a high protein intake (primarily animal proteins) is associated with increased cancer, diabetes, and overall mortality.[18] However, in subjects over the age of 65, higher dietary protein was found to be protective. This discrepancy in itself makes no sense. How can higher animal protein consumption *increase* the cancer death risk from ages 50 – 65 but then miraculously *reduce* cancer mortality at age 65 and beyond? But regardless of the initial claim, association does not mean causation. Moreover, a veritable who's who in protein research critiqued the observational study in a "Letter to the

Editor" in the journal *Cell Metabolism*. Though the journal refused to publish the letter, the scientists wrote,[19]

> *"...The study design and analyses are inappropriate; key contradictory data are neglected; and conclusions are not justified by the data. As scientists with decades of experience studying the impact of protein on health, we are concerned that translation of these flawed data and exaggerated conclusions to the public could have serious negative health consequences for adults seeking to maintain muscle health and avoid sarcopenia."*

In their letter entitled "The Contrived Association of Dietary Protein with Mortality," the protein experts made the following incredible observation:

> *"In their study, Levine et al. indicate (Figure 1, Table S1, and Discussion) that '...the level of protein is ... not associated with differences in all-cause, cancer, or CVD mortality.' In fact, the data demonstrate that cancer mortality was actually ~10% higher in the low protein group compared with the higher protein group (i.e., 9.8% versus 9.0% deaths). We would argue that these obvious findings are the most important."*

Rather than relying on biased and flawed epidemiological studies, let's take an evidence-based look at the safety and tremendous health benefits of animal protein.

Meat Is What Made Us Human

Over the past 2 million years, the brain size of our prehuman ancestors increased rapidly and dramatically to become roughly three times the size of other primate brains.[20] At the same time, a nearly identical reduction in the size of the human gastrointestinal tract also occurred. According to a theory called the "expensive tissue hypothesis," the increased energy demands of the relatively large human brain are balanced by a corresponding reduction in the size of the equally metabolically expensive (i.e., high-energy-consuming) gut. A shift in gut *proportions* also took place. More than half of the human gut volume (56%) is dominated by the small intestine—it's the main site of nutrient absorption and digestion—whereas the colon makes up only about 20% of the gut. In contrast, the chimp gut is dominated by the colon (greater than 50%).[21] These changes in gut size and proportion are important to keep in mind as we discuss major dietary changes that transpired during the same evolutionary period.

The anatomy and physiology of digestive systems in animals has evolved in concert with their diets. Herbivores are ideally suited to digesting and absorbing carbohydrate foods. To digest plant matter, they have evolved enlarged and/or elongated digestive tracts to compensate for the formidable process of breaking down the cellulose in plant cell walls. The large guts of herbivores contain fermentation vats where fibrous food is retained for prolonged periods to allow for maximal exposure to microbial digestion, resulting in the production of short-chain fatty acids as a major energy source.[22]

The vast majority of foods eaten by primates come from plant sources. Gorillas and orangutans eat almost exclusively plant foods (99%), while the largely fruit-based diet of chimpanzees checks in at being 87% – 98% plant-sourced. However, the nutritional quality of bulky plant matter such as insoluble fiber and seeds pales in comparison to animal foods that are nutrient- and energy-dense as well as highly digestible. As the planet became cooler and drier during the Ice Ages, our prehuman ancestors switched from a primarily plant-centered diet to one that routinely incorporated animal-sourced foods as well. This is partly evidenced by the discovery of early stone tools alongside the fossilized remains of early humans. Stone tools were used to carve flesh from animal remains and pry marrow out of their bones. Fossilized bones of animals bearing cut marks made by stone tools provide further proof that humans were avid meat-eaters.[21]

Are We *Hypercarnivores?*

In a groundbreaking study published in 2021 in the *Yearbook of Physical Anthropology* (published by the American Association of Biological Anthropologists), Dr. Miki Ben-Dor and his colleagues at Tel Aviv University reconstructed the diet of Paleolithic humans based not on comparisons of present-day hunter-gatherer communities, but rather on evidence stemming from human biology and archaeology. This evidence was derived from about 400 research papers stemming from a variety of scientific fields. The study authors showed that humans possess various physical and behavioral traits that place us in the carnivore fraternity. For example, we have a higher stomach acidity level than omnivores and even other predators do. Since stomach acid serves partly as a natural antiseptic, high stomach acidity likely evolved because of high pathogen levels linked to bacteria-laden old meat that was consumed over several days or weeks.

In contrast to the universal assumption that the survival of early humans was attributable to their capacity to eat *both* animals and plants, this unprecedented review of studies concluded that humans evolved at the top of the food chain as "apex predators." Since they derived 70% of their food from animals, Paleolithic humans were considered *hypercarnivores*. They did consume plant foods as well, but plant contributions to their diet only became significant towards the end of the Stone Age era, when the availability of animal foods diminished coincident with the extinction of larger animals.

Bottom line: the scientific reality is that humans evolved as consumers of **protein** and **fat** rather than carbohydrates.

Regular consumption of high-quality animal foods allowed for the natural selection of a large, energy-consuming brain and a smaller colon linked to a longer small intestine. This arrangement made humans better suited to handle a nutritionally dense, highly digestible diet that included substantially fewer bulky, fibrous, and otherwise indigestible components. Without habitually including animal foods in their diet, in all likelihood, our prehuman ancestors would *not* have evolved into modern humans with large and complex brains.[21]

It's worth noting that one line of human ancestors—the *Paranthropus* species—continued a dietary trajectory of eating mostly plant foods during the Ice Ages. However, due to shifts in climate, they had to sustain themselves on lower-quality fallback foods such as bark and unripe fruit. In the end, *Paranthropus* did not do well and became extinct.[21] In contrast, the *Homo* species thrived on an increasingly carnivorous diet.

But how exactly did animal foods enable the phenomenal growth of our ancestors' brains and make us human? Simple. *Meat: it's what's for dinner!*

The brain is the fattiest organ in the body, clocking in at nearly 60% fat. The two most abundant polyunsaturated fats in the brain, DHA (docosahexaenoic acid) and ARA (arachidonic acid), rapidly accumulate in the infant brain during the first years of life. These long-chain fatty acids play essential structural and functional roles as constituents of cell membranes and are important for brain development during both the fetal and postnatal periods. Infant formula fortified with DHA and ARA has been shown to enhance cognitive development.[23]

Normal nerve function cannot occur without DHA and ARA. For our prehuman ancestors, muscle meat was a good source of ARA, whereas fish and scavenged brain tissue provided a generous supply of both ARA *and* DHA. Scavenged bone marrow was an especially concentrated source of the high-in-fat calories that were required to meet the high-energy demands of the evolving and growing brain. Plants, in contrast, contain little or no DHA and ARA. While plants do provide precursor fatty acids (linoleic acid and alpha-linolenic acid) to be used for the synthesis of DHA and ARA, this process is inefficient. Interestingly, compared with the herbivores they devour, carnivores have a proportionately larger brain relative to their body size. *The evolution of the carnivore brain—i.e., the brains of our early ancestors—resulted from the consumption of animal tissues (meat, fish, and organs) that provided key structural components such as DHA and ARA that are necessary for brain growth.* Conversely, evolutionary brain development (enlargement) in herbivores may have been thwarted by the limited internal production of DHA and ARA from plant food and by the absence of these fatty acids in grass, leaves, and other plant materials the herbivores regularly consumed.[24]

Meat, fish, and organs are concentrated sources of many important vitamins, minerals, and essential fatty acids that humans need, such as vitamin B12, vitamin D, preformed vitamin A, vitamin K2, iron, calcium, zinc, and choline. All of these are essential nutrients that are either missing in or poorly absorbed from plant foods.

Vitamin B12, zinc, and choline are particularly vital for brain development. That's because the synthesis of new DNA is essential for rapid cell division and growth in the developing fetus and brain. This process requires vitamin B12—without it, nerve damage and brain atrophy can occur.[25] Since meat, dairy, and other animal foods are our primary dietary sources of vitamin B12, an individual eating a diet of exclusively plant foods runs the risk of having a B12 deficiency. Vitamin B12 is not found in plant foods. Some algae contain tiny amounts of *pseudo*vitamin B12, but these so-called "B12 analogues" are inactive in humans.[26] In a study of 107 volunteers aged 61 to 87 years, brain volume loss was associated with low vitamin B12 status.[27] *Could low vitamin B12 status have contributed to the shrinkage of our human brain over the last 10,000 years, a* *period that coincided with the advent of agriculture and humans consequently consuming a greater proportion of plant foods?*[28]

Next to iron, zinc is the most abundant mineral in the body. Zinc is required for the activation of over 300 enzymes and more than 1,000 transcription factors (proteins that transcribe DNA into RNA). These requirements are a clear indication of the vital importance that zinc has for our health.[29] In particular, zinc activates key enzymes in the developing brain while also maintaining brain function in adults. Low zinc status has been associated with impaired brain development and implicated in neurodegenerative disorders such as Alzheimer's disease.[30] Plant-based diets contain high levels of phytic acid, an anti-nutrient that binds to zinc (and many other essential minerals) in our GI tracts. Phytic acid significantly reduces how much zinc we can absorb from all foods, even zinc-rich red meat and other animal foods—we can absorb much more zinc if we don't simultaneously also eat foods that contain phytic acid.[31] According to a systematic review of multiple studies and a meta-analysis, vegetarians have low zinc intakes and low zinc status.[32]

Although not as well-known as B12 and zinc, choline is a vital yet overlooked nutrient that plays central roles in fat metabolism, liver function, brain and neurological development (it's a precursor for the body's synthesis of acetylcholine, a neurotransmitter that facilitates learning and memory), and gene expression. Dietary intake is essential since the amount produced in the body is not sufficient to support body needs. However, most people living in North America, Europe, and Australia are not meeting their choline requirements. A deficiency of choline has been linked to liver disease, neural tube defects during pregnancy, and other neurological disorders. Since choline is predominantly found in animal foods (e.g., eggs, meat, seafood, and dairy products), the growing (and disturbing) trend towards plant-based diets with less meat consumption could lead to even greater shortcomings in choline intake/status. Indeed, research using NHANES 2009-2014 datasets suggests that without eating eggs (the richest food source next to liver) or taking a supplement, it is extremely difficult to get enough choline.[33]

Interestingly, although beef is commonly associated with saturated fat, the most plentiful fatty acid in beef is actually oleic acid,[34] the exact same health-promoting monounsaturated fatty acid found in high amounts in olive oil, avocado, and nuts! Whereas dietary saturated fat is generally neutral (i.e., not harmful), oleic acid has cardioprotective and anti-aging properties. Studies have shown that oleic acid lowers LDL cholesterol and may increase beneficial HDL. Oleic acid also induces a shift from small, dense LDL to large, buoyant LDL. The small LDL particles more easily penetrate the artery wall lining, promoting the formation of fatty plaques that can lead to atherosclerosis. In contrast, the larger particles have not been shown to be atherogenic (capable of promoting fatty plaques in arteries).[35] With regard to anti-aging effects, a review of randomized clinical trials determined that oleic acid is a natural activator of SIRT1, a sirtuin protein linked to increased longevity (see Chapter 7).[36]

Oddly, the emergence of animal foods into the human diet allowed us to consume more undesirable plant foods that were lower in nutritional quality and potentially harmful. For example, while cassava root is a rich source of calories, it contains chemical compounds called "cyanogenic glycosides." These chemicals serve as a natural defense mechanism to protect the plant from being eaten by herbivores and insects, thus allowing it to survive and produce offspring. In humans, however, cassava root releases poisonous cyanide into the body if the root has not been properly processed by fermentation, cooking, and drying to reduce the cyanide content to tolerable and safe levels. Meanwhile, animal foods provide high-quality protein, particularly sulfur-containing amino acids such as cysteine and methionine. These amino acids are essential for the detoxification of cyanide. Because plants are relatively low in these sulfuric amino acids, incorporating animal proteins in their diet enabled our ancestors to eat energy-rich but potentially noxious plant foods they otherwise would have passed up.[21]

Today, many people across the globe rely on plants such as cassava as important sources of calories. However, in the case of people in developing countries, these populations also suffer from protein deficiency, which impairs cyanide detoxification. Thus, a major concern is that people eating poorly processed cassava root are at high risk for cyanide-induced neuropathy. Furthermore, a cassava-based diet *without sufficient animal protein* may adversely affect children's growth and development.[37]

All in all, our prehuman ancestors would have needed a smaller amount of more nutrient-dense animal food compared with copious amounts of much-less-nutrient-dense plant food to satisfy their nutritional requirements. Similar to how our physiology adapted to a highly physically active lifestyle, we also acquired a larger brain and smaller gut as we transitioned to consuming more animal foods. But as previously mentioned, the later decline in the quality of our nutrition that coincided with the dawn of agriculture during the Neolithic period may have led to our human brain shrinking.

The Myth That Meat Causes Chronic Disease

In recent years, we have been bombarded with incessant fearmongering insisting that eating meat is harmful to our health. Books, magazines, and blatantly biased documentary films use clever scare tactics to make us believe that meat causes heart disease, colon cancer, diabetes, and Alzheimer's disease. As I will discuss in this section, these melodramatic claims are not supported by any direct scientific evidence.

Unfortunately, the axiom that "A lie repeated often enough becomes accepted truth" very much applies to this issue. Today, the popular perception—which, again, is emphatically not true—is that meat is unhealthy for us and bad for the environment and thus should be avoided or limited. Likewise, veganism is perceived to be so "healthful" that people who are unable to achieve this level of dietary extremism actually believe they are *less* healthy because of their lack of resolve—they believe they just don't have what it takes to reach such a "pinnacle of health." More often than not, entrepreneurs who appear on the popular television show *Shark Tank* seeking investments for a novel food product boast that their invention is vegan. Well, of course! It's a smart marketing decision.

Regrettably, the irrational notion that shunning all animal food is good for our health is a misguided perception that's held by a growing number of American consumers. But the crazy notion that meat and other animal foods cause cancer and other diseases runs counter to human evolution! *Should we throw out the very food that spurred the growth of our brains and made us human? Really?*

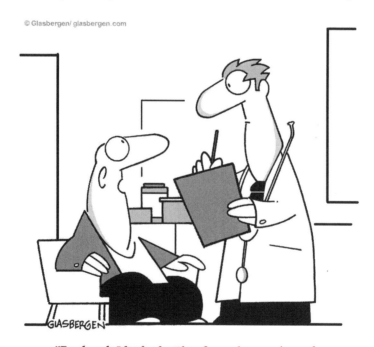

© Glasbergen/ glasbergen.com

"For lunch I had a bottle of root beer, a bag of potato chips and two candy bars. Giving up red meat is easier than I thought!"

When discussing nutrition research, it is absolutely paramount to first distinguish between *interventional studies* and *observational epidemiology*. Interventional studies are designed to evaluate the effect of a specific treatment or preventive measure on outcomes by randomly assigning participants to either the interventional group or a control (placebo) group. Ideally, this is carried out as a randomized double-blind, placebo-controlled trial wherein both the researchers and the participants are unaware of the assigned intervention. As mentioned in Chapter 4, randomized clinical trials (RCTs) are considered the gold standard for research. Nevertheless, interventional studies are infrequently done due to the great deal of work and expense that's required to conduct them.

Most nutrition research involves observational analyses of large groups of people over long periods, either going forward (prospectively) or looking to the past (retrospectively). The aim of these types of studies is to identify associations between dietary variables and health effects. This is typically done using food frequency questionnaires. There is no intervention. At best, observational epidemiology merely shows correlations—they do not show causation. This glaring shortcoming of epidemiology can easily be illustrated by a hypothetical study showing that people who ski have a higher prevalence of psoriasis. Does this mean that skiing causes psoriasis? Of course not. It is merely a correlation. Correlation does not equal causation. Consider also that preliminary results from a *real* study published in the scientific literature showed that being born under the Leo sign is associated with a higher risk of dying.[38] Need I say more? But I will.

Nutrition observational studies are fraught with confounding factors. One of those is the use of food frequency questionnaires. Most people simply cannot accurately recall what they were eating several months ago. Can you? And so these food questionnaires do not reflect absolute intakes—they only approximate past eating behaviors. Also, study participants often overestimate their consumption of fruits and vegetables. This is partly due to social desirability bias, which is to say they report eating foods that are perceived to be healthier (read: more socially acceptable) instead of what they *actually* eat.[39]

The most challenging confounding factor in nutrition epidemiology is what's known as the "healthy user bias." Observational studies showing improved health outcomes resulting from eating a plant-based diet can only demonstrate a correlation, not causation. Since a plant-based diet is *perceived* to be healthy, people following such a diet typically practice other healthy behaviors, like exercising, managing their stress, getting restful sleep, and/or meditating. They are also less inclined to smoke, drink, or regularly eat processed foods and sugar. Conversely, observational studies that incriminate meat for causing disease do not control for the "unhealthy user bias," which is the opposite cohort. In this instance, study subjects who are habitual meat eaters tend to practice unhealthy behaviors such as smoking, drinking, and eating junk food. Just as pursuing an overall healthy lifestyle probably accounts for the benefits of plant-based eating—*not* the diet itself—an unhealthy lifestyle and the absence of healthy behaviors are likely to blame for the ill effects associated with meat consumption.

Finally, to further illustrate the futility of these observational studies, recent systematic reviews of observational studies found that *nearly all foods* were significantly associated with either an increased or decreased risk of dying.[40] According to Dr. John Ioannidis, esteemed Stanford University professor, research critic, and author of the celebrated paper "Why Most Published Research Findings are False"[41]:

> *"Almost all nutritional variables are correlated with one another; thus, if one variable is causally related to health outcomes, many other variables will also yield significant associations in large enough data sets. With more research*

involving big data, almost all nutritional variables will be associated with almost all outcomes. Moreover, given the complicated associations of eating behaviors and patterns with many time-varying social and behavioral factors that also affect health, no currently available cohort includes sufficient information to address confounding in nutritional association."

With the understanding that associations of nutritional factors are often misconstrued by the media and ergo the public as being a direct cause and effect, let us now take a critical look at the research on the supposed meat-disease connection.

Meat and Cancer

According to the 2015 – 2020 Dietary Guidelines for Americans, we should limit consumption of red meat (including processed meats) to about one serving *per week*. That's about 3.5 ounces of cooked meat, which is roughly the size of a deck of cards.[42] Also in 2015, the World Health Organization International Agency for Research on Cancer branded red meat as "probably carcinogenic" to humans and placed processed meats in a category - "carcinogenic to humans" - that also includes cigarettes.[43] Not surprisingly, these recommendations were predicated on weak evidence gleaned from flawed *observational* studies. Moreover, the bulk of these studies (about 76%) linking red and processed meats to cancer involved people in Western countries. In contrast, most of the studies conducted in Asian populations showed that consumption of red and processed meats is *not* associated with the onset of cancer.[44] These inconsistent findings suggest that factors other than meat are the real suspects. Do you recall the ridiculous headline "Diets High in Meat, Eggs, and Dairy Could Be as Harmful to Health as Smoking" in *The Guardian*? This article was nothing more than grandstanding. Is it logical to believe that high-quality animal foods that we thrived on for millennia are suddenly just as damaging to our health as a substance filled with hundreds of known carcinogens?

Notably, four systematic reviews (including both randomized trials and observational studies) recently performed by an independent consortium of researchers from seven countries addressed the current evidence vilifying the consumption of red meat and processed meat.[45] Collectively, the comprehensive reviews concluded that the certainty of evidence for the potential harmful effects (and the degree of effects) of meat consumption was low to exceptionally low. The panel of researchers therefore recommended that people *continue rather than reduce* their consumption of unprocessed red meat and processed meat. And this despite the fact that most of the studies assessed were of the low-quality observational type! The panel members stated:

> *"These recommendations are, however, primarily based on observational studies that are at high risk for confounding and thus are limited in establishing causal inferences, nor do they report the absolute magnitude of any possible effects. Furthermore, the organizations that produce guidelines did not conduct or access rigorous systematic reviews of the evidence, were limited in addressing conflicts of interest, and did not explicitly address population values and preferences, raising questions regarding adherence to guideline standards for trustworthiness."*

Not surprisingly, since the seemingly controversial findings from this study challenged the incessant anti-meat narrative we so often hear, saying that meat does *not* cause us harm had the plant-based universe up in arms.

Meat and Heart Disease

Apart from the cancer concern, another major issue frequently raised about red meat is that it's rich in saturated fat. For decades, dietary saturated fat—the kind that's usually solid at room temperature—has been villainized as a cause of cardiovascular disease (CVD). The current U.S. Dietary Guidelines recommend that we limit our intake of saturated fat to no more than 10% of our calories to lower our CVD risk. However, more recent evidence from meta-analyses of randomized clinical trials as well as observational studies do *not* support such a restriction of dietary saturated fat. These studies show no significant association between saturated fat intake and CVD or risk of death.[46] For example, the landmark PURE study involving 135,000 people from 18 countries on five continents demonstrated that increased consumption of all types of fat (including saturated fat) correlated with lower mortality and had a neutral association with CVD. Notably, this large study showed that those who consumed the most saturated fat (at roughly 14% of their total daily calories) had a *decreased* risk of stroke, a finding supported by previous meta-analyses of multiple studies.[47,48]

It's important to understand that while the saturated fat we eat is not associated with chronic disease based on the overwhelming evidence cited here, higher levels of specific types of saturated fatty acids in the bloodstream *do* increase the risk of metabolic syndrome, diabetes, CVD, heart failure, and premature death. However, *blood levels* of saturated fatty acids are not related to *dietary* saturated fat—they actually correlate closely with dietary carbohydrates, meaning that when we eat carbohydrates, *that's* when our blood levels of saturated fatty acids go up. In fact, increasing our intake of saturated fat two- to threefold may even lower our circulating levels of saturated fatty acids *if we also eat fewer carbohydrates*. This occurs because a low-carbohydrate diet enhances the burning of fat for fuel—with a preference for saturated fatty acids—while *also* reducing the production of fat in the liver from carbs.[46] According to the PURE study, a higher consumption of carbohydrates from starches and sugars and *not* a higher consumption of saturated fat is what increases the risk of CVD and death.[47,48]

When consumed to replace carbohydrates or unsaturated fatty acids in the diet, saturated fatty acids can raise levels of LDL cholesterol. (Unsaturated fatty acids are usually liquid at room temperature; we think of them as oils.) It's true that LDL cholesterol contributes to the development of CVD. However, the elevation in LDL cholesterol caused by consuming saturated fat is primarily due to an increase in large, fluffy LDL particles, and these have a substantially *weaker* association with CVD risk than smaller, dense LDL particles do. That's because compared with their larger counterparts, the smaller, more tightly packed particles can more easily penetrate the artery wall and form plaques. Overconsumption of carbohydrates, *not* saturated fat, is linked to increased small LDL particles. What's more, cutting back on saturated fat *lowers* levels of beneficial HDL particles. Ultimately, the effects of increased dietary saturated fat on CVD risk are not accurately evidenced by elevated levels of LDL cholesterol.[46]

Additional proof that the saturated fat in meat does not promote heart disease lies in the finding that processed meat *is* linked to increased CVD risk, while unprocessed red meat is *not*. This despite the fact that both contain saturated fat.[49] Incidentally, we humans have an innate preference for dietary fat that dates back to our Paleolithic ancestors—they primarily hunted large, fatty animals and transported fatty parts such as fat-rich bone marrow to a central location.[50]

Meat and Child Development

In recent years, beef consumption in the U.S. has actually declined over 14% due in part to misinformation about protein and fat in meats.[51] In an interview with *AgriLife Today*, Dr. Guoyao Wu, distinguished professor in the Department of Animal Science at Texas A&M University, raised concern about adverse effects resulting from limited or no consumption of meat and other animal-sourced proteins, particularly among growing children:[52]

"People on a vegan diet tend to forget how important high-quality protein is to human growth and health... If you look at the population of some Asian countries, most males are short and the children are stunted. Twenty years ago, one-third of the children were stunted. Now, less than 10% are stunted because of increased consumption of animal-sourced protein in their diets... Children especially need meat to build skeletal muscle... They are at a critical stage in their lives as their bodies continue to develop and mature. Without sufficient sources of protein, their muscle, bones, and other organs will not develop properly, which will lead to health problems later in life...If you look at some countries, children are stunted. They have primarily a corn-based diet. Corn contains so little amino acids compared with meat. When I see stunted children or adults in the U.S. due to limited or no consumption of animal protein, I feel very sad...Our country has the greatest abundance of protein, but some choose to live such an unhealthy lifestyle."

Meat Is a Functional Food

Beyond the fact that meat is a superior source of high-quality protein and essential vitamins and minerals not found in plant foods, meat is also considered to be a "functional food." Functional foods are foods that promote health and help prevent disease in a manner that extends beyond their nutritional impact. Coffee, green tea, and olive oil are examples of functional foods that naturally contain bioactive compounds that contribute to the prevention of chronic diseases like cancer and heart disease by exerting antioxidant and anti-inflammatory effects.[53]

In Chapter 5, we talked about the health benefits of four nonessential though physiologically important nutrients—carnosine, creatine, taurine, and anserine—that are especially abundant in beef but absent in plants. (Even the precursors of these nutrients are low in most plant proteins.) Some of these amino acids and dipeptides (two amino acids linked together) are also referred to as "functional" amino acids because they regulate key metabolic pathways to improve health, a function that goes beyond protein synthesis.[54] Another important functional amino acid found in beef but lacking in plants is hydroxyproline, which is a major constituent of collagen. Clinical studies have shown that supplementation with hydroxyproline-containing collagen peptides markedly improves skin, joint, and bone health.

All in all, these five functional nutrients have tremendous health-promoting effects, including the potential to boost immune defenses to counter infections by pathogenic bacteria, fungi, parasites, and viruses, including the coronavirus. As a rich source of these nutrients, beef can certainly be classified as being a functional food.[54]

The Myth That Meat Is Bad for the Environment

A major driver of climate change is the generation of greenhouse gases, primarily carbon dioxide, methane, and nitrous oxide. These gases accumulate in our atmosphere and trap heat from the sun, thus making the planet warmer. In 2006, the United Nations Food and Agricultural Organization (FAO) released a report claiming that rearing cattle produces more global warming greenhouse gases than transportation as a category does. The report contends that domestic animals are responsible for 18% of all greenhouse gas emissions.[55] But according to University of California–Davis Professor Frank Mitloehner, an air quality scientist and an authority on farming and greenhouse gases, the statements regarding the contribution of livestock to climate change are inaccurate and highly overstated.[56]

One major error in the report involves a complete life-cycle assessment that adds up all of the emissions from every phase of production in a particular industry. Mitloehner points out that the FAO's life-cycle analysis of livestock production takes into account both direct and indirect emissions that encompass all gases produced from the farm to the table, e.g., gases released from gut fermentation, manure, growing animal feed, and processing meat and dairy foods. On the other hand, the transportation assessment only considers direct (tailpipe) emissions from the burning of fossil fuels. It overlooks other sources of emissions such as the production of car/plane parts, the transportation of parts to factories, and the deterioration and weathering of roads and runways.[56,57] In short, this is a classic example of comparing apples to oranges.

In particular, the FAO's claims about methane emissions from livestock are greatly exaggerated. Methane from belching cows is not a major player in the methane concentration in the atmosphere. According to new calculations by NASA, the sharp increase in methane emissions since 2006 has come from the oil and gas industry, fires, and microbial production in wet tropical environments (e.g., marshes and rice paddies).[58]

We need to distinguish between fossil-fuel-derived carbon emissions and nature's carbon cycle wherein carbon flows from the atmosphere to the Earth and then back into the atmosphere. Combustion of fossil fuel is the primary contributor to the high concentration of atmospheric carbon because it adds an amount of *new* carbon dioxide to the atmosphere that exceeds the capacity of plants, soils, and oceans to capture and store it. Conversely, methane (carbon) produced by livestock is equal to the amount of methane sequestered, provided that the numbers of livestock remain constant. In fact, livestock-induced GHGs (greenhouse gases) in developed nations are approaching a plateau and even decreasing because livestock numbers have remained unchanged.[57] In developing countries, however, increasing numbers of livestock are causing accompanying GHGs to rise. Even so, methane gas is short-lived—it only stays in the atmosphere for a decade, after which time it's broken down to water vapor and carbon dioxide as part of the natural carbon cycle. In contrast, carbon dioxide has a half-life of 1,000 years! The FAO and the International Atomic Energy Agency published a report in 2003 addressing the issue of methane emissions from ruminants (e.g., cattle, sheep)[59]:

"Prior to 1999, there was a strong relationship between the change in atmospheric methane concentrations and the world ruminant populations. However, since 1999, this strong relation has disappeared. This change in relationship between the atmosphere and ruminant numbers suggests that the role of ruminants in greenhouse gases may be less significant than originally thought, with other sources and sinks playing a larger role in global methane accounting."

It's worth noting that 70% of all agricultural land on the planet is suitable *only for ruminant livestock production, not crop production.* As part of nature's carbon cycle (see diagram below), cattle actually benefit our climate by trapping and storing carbon from the atmosphere through the consumption of carbon-rich plants. Cattle and other livestock ruminants convert energy-dense but nutrient-poor plant material that humans can't eat—grasses and forage—into nutrient-dense meat and dairy products. These products provide us with high-quality protein and key nutrients that are not obtainable from plants.[57] Manure from livestock directly increases the amount of carbon in the soil while also improving soil quality to promote the growth of carbon-dioxide-trapping plants. (Remarkably, soil stores three times more carbon than the atmosphere does.) An enormous amount of carbon is thus sequestered in the ground, offsetting methane from cow burps and resulting in lowered total GHG emissions or even a net GHG reduction.[60]

Importantly, this environmentally beneficial soil sequestration of carbon pertains to cattle grazing on pasture over the entire life cycle. According to a meta-analysis, grazing lands sequester and store enough of a surplus of carbon to offset rural GHG emissions, and could even completely or partially cancel out emissions from urban areas as well.[61] Thus, 100% grass-fed beef is environmentally superior to beef from feedlots, also known as concentrated animal feeding operations (CAFO). Unlike grazing lands, these CAFO facilities confine large numbers (thousands) of animals in close proximity.

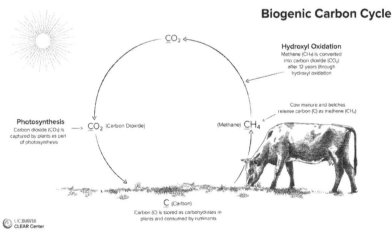

Biogenic Carbon Cycle

CO_2

Hydroxyl Oxidation
Methane (CH_4) is converted into carbon dioxide (CO_2) after 12 years through hydroxyl oxidation

Cow manure and belches release carbon (C) as methane (CH_4)

Photosynthesis
Carbon dioxide (CO_2) is captured by plants as part of photosynthesis

CO_2 (Carbon Dioxide)

(Methane) CH_4

C (Carbon)
Carbon (C) is stored as carbohydrates in plants and consumed by ruminants

UCDAVIS
CLEAR Center

In the U.S., advancements in animal agriculture have led to producing more food with less GHG production. Greater reproductive efficiency, improved veterinary care, cutting-edge breeding techniques, and better feeding practices (e.g., food that's more calorie-dense) have all contributed to the world's historically lowest carbon footprint per unit of animal-sourced food production. Globally, improved food production efficiency is needed to meet the increasing demand for animal-sourced foods from growing populations.[57]

Based on a simulated system, eliminating all animal agriculture and animal-derived foods in the U.S. would result in a paltry **2.6%** reduction in GHG emissions.[62] The U.S. Environmental Protection Agency (EPA) reports that *all livestock (beef, dairy, swine, and poultry) together contribute only 4.2% of GHGs.*[63] Despite this truth, the media and activists continue to promulgate the highly inflated 18% figure from the FAO, steering us in the wrong direction toward a more plant-centered diet with fewer animal-sourced foods. Such a misguided attempt at achieving a supposedly sustainable diet would lead to an overall increase in the consumption of calories and carbohydrates, more damaging deficiencies of nutrients such as vitamin B12 and EPA/DHA omega-3 fatty acids, and a large portion of our agricultural land being unavailable for human use. Instead of reducing meat and dairy consumption, the focus should clearly be on scaling back the use of fossil fuels, which are the main contributors to global warming. According to the EPA, around 80% of all GHGs emanate from transportation, industry, and power.[63]

"The notion that a change of diet would have a drastic impact on climate is completely overblown, and in my opinion, quite dangerous," says Dr. Mitloehner. "It takes our attention from where that 800-pound gorilla sits, and that's square in the area of fossil fuels."[64]

Consider that in 1800, the U.S. had around 80 million ruminate animals (buffalo) and no cars or trucks. Today, there are approximately 90 million cattle in the U.S. and more than 260 million vehicles on highways.[65] That pretty much says it all!

To add to the adverse outcomes previously noted, shifting to a more plant-based diet diminishes the quantity and quality of protein in the diet, increasing the risk of amino acid deficiencies. Contrary to plant-based propaganda, plants fed to beef and dairy cattle are unfit for human consumption and thus cannot be used as protein sources. Plant-centered diets would lower our average daily protein intake to only 50 – 60 grams/day. Though this range of dietary protein satisfies the RDA, considerable evidence from research studies shows that protein intakes of *more than 100 grams/day* enhance muscle and metabolic health and optimize overall adult health. As for protein quality, ruminants such as cattle convert poor-quality protein from grasses, hay, and corn silage that we cannot eat into superior high-quality animal protein that provides us with the optimal balance of essential amino acids. Currently, more than one-third of the planet's protein is provided by livestock.[65] Dr. Donald Layman, Professor Emeritus of Nutrition at the University of Illinois and a world-renowned protein researcher, points out that recommendations made regarding lessening the impact of agriculture on the environment should also emphasize the optimal utilization of natural resources to create healthful diets that meet the world's protein needs[65]:

"Sustainable production of protein needs to be a foundation of a sustainable diet, and livestock have a critical role in production of high-quality protein."

For a much more extensive discussion on the topic of meat consumption, see the Appendix for two phenomenal books: *Sacred*

Cow by Diana Rogers and Robb Wolf and *The Carnivore Code* by Paul Saladino.

Anti-Meat Propaganda

The anti-meat hysteria never ends, unfortunately. In early 2022, public schools in New York City started serving meat-free vegan meals on Fridays. This totally unnecessary initiative by the city's Department of Education only furthers the baseless (and strange) perception that the most nutritious human food on the planet will kill us. Sadly, children will be brainwashed into thinking that eating meat is unhealthy. As it is, Americans derive 70% of their total daily calories from plant-based foods.[66] Perhaps the plant-based crusaders are unaware that—unlike cows and giraffes—we humans do not have large fermentation vats in our guts and cannot digest plant-based foods as efficiently as ruminants can.

The plant-based movement is also touting fake meat and "meat" created in a lab as suitable alternatives. The authors of a study using metabolomics (the practice of measuring metabolites) to determine how plant-based mock burgers stack up against real burgers concluded that "a plant burger is not really a beef burger."[67] The study, published in *Scientific Reports*, found that 171 out of 190 metabolites differed between real beef and a plant-based meat alternative even though the nutrition panels were similar. Creatine, DHA, hydroxyproline, and anserine were among the 22 metabolites only found in beef. While DHA is an essential omega-3 fatty acid particularly important for brain and heart health, the other metabolites are functional nutrients with profound health-promoting effects such as anti-inflammatory and immunomodulatory activities (see Chapter 5).

Moreover, plant-based fake meats are often loaded with low-quality legume or grain proteins such as soy protein isolate and wheat gluten. In contrast with fermented soy foods, soy protein isolate is a heavily processed powder rich in phytoestrogens as well as anti-nutrients such as phytic acid. (Again, phytic acid can impede the absorption of critical minerals such as zinc and iron.) Wheat gluten is an irritant to the gut lining even in people without celiac disease and may lead to adverse health effects in susceptible individuals. In addition, large amounts of highly unstable corn oil are also present in many fake meat products. Polyunsaturated seed oils such as corn oil are known to promote the development of cancer in lab animals.[68] *Do we really need to increase our consumption of ultra-processed plant-based fake meats laden with soy protein isolate, wheat gluten, and corn oil, among other noxious additives?* While our own health will surely not benefit from eating this garbage, the CEOs and venture capitalists who fund these inferior processed junk foods will most definitely profit.

What About Eggs and Dairy?

The fact that the cholesterol-rich egg does not elevate serum cholesterol levels for most people should be common knowledge by now. The 2015 U.S. Dietary Guidelines for Americans state that **"cholesterol is no longer considered a nutrient of concern for overconsumption"** among healthy adults.[69] Not only is increased egg consumption *not* correlated with a higher risk of CVD, it may in fact be linked to a *decreased* risk of stroke![46] In addition, numerous studies have shown that higher dietary cholesterol is associated with *lower* levels of small, dense LDL particles (plaque-forming) and *higher* levels of large, buoyant LDL particles (weakly linked to CVD risk) as well as protective HDL particles.[70]

We cannot survive without cholesterol—it is in every cell in our bodies. Cholesterol is required primarily to build cell membranes, produce hormones (e.g., estrogen, testosterone, cortisol), make vitamin D, and produce bile to break down fats during digestion.

Egg protein is of such high quality that its amino acid composition is used as the gold standard against which all other proteins are compared. Eggs are also one of the richest sources of sulfur amino acids (e.g., methionine, cysteine) that are used to make glutathione, the body's master antioxidant and detoxifier.[71] In short, eggs are a powerhouse of nutrition! They're loaded with vitamins and minerals such as vitamin B12, vitamin D, vitamin A, vitamin E, folate (vitamin B9), riboflavin (vitamin B2), iron, zinc, and selenium. They also contain lutein and zeaxanthin, important pigments that protect our eyes from harmful UV rays. Importantly, *all of these nutrients are found in the egg yolk*, so please eat the whole egg!

Interestingly, the bioavailability of the dietary carotenoids lutein and zeaxanthin in egg yolks is significantly higher than what green leafy vegetables offer.[72] (Perhaps Mother Nature is trying to tell us something?) We can much better absorb these carotenoids from egg yolks because yolks also contain a high number of fat-like molecules called "phospholipids" that facilitate the uptake of carotenoids into cell membranes. Yolks also contain other lipids that enhance carotenoid absorption. Among those lipids are triglycerides and...wait for it...*cholesterol!*

Let's move on to dairy, another food that's often maligned as being an "inflammatory" food. However, that's just another myth, one that's often aided and abetted by vegan advocates and companies that stand to financially gain from consumers ditching dairy products. According to three reviews of randomized clinical trials, dairy foods *do not* show a pro-inflammatory effect in healthy subjects or individuals with metabolic disorders (e.g., obese adults). In fact, dairy has significant *anti-inflammatory* properties.[73-75] And why wouldn't it? After all, maternal milk supports the development of the infant's immune system, curbs the growth of bacteria, and provides antioxidant protection.

Like eggs, dairy foods are packed with calcium, magnesium, vitamin B12, and many other bioavailable essential nutrients. And high-quality dairy protein is a phenomenal muscle builder! Furthermore, recent evidence indicates that consumption of dairy fat is associated with a significantly lower risk of type 2 diabetes.[76] Dairy fat consists of an assortment of diverse types of saturated fatty acids. In particular, a dairy fat called *trans*-palmitoleic acid appears to be most closely linked to a reduced risk of diabetes. In addition, the fat in cheese (which contributes a large portion of most people's dairy fat consumption) is a rich source of vitamin K2. Vitamin K2 improves insulin secretion and insulin sensitivity and thus may also play a role in lowering the risk of diabetes.[77]

Despite all of this, some people argue against eating dairy foods because of certain peptides (protein fragments) in milk that demonstrate opioid (morphine-like) activity. One of these peptides, beta-casomorphine-7 (BCM7), has been linked to adverse health effects, including an increased risk of cardiovascular diseases and type 1 diabetes.[78] Conversely, other studies have shown that these dairy-derived beta-casomorphins provide health *benefits* by reducing inflammation, oxidative stress, and kidney damage caused by diabetes.[79,80] In any case, an extensive review of studies failed to find any strong evidence of a cause-and-effect relationship between BCM7 (or any other similar peptides) and the development of any chronic disease such as CVD or type 1 diabetes.[81] Moreover, the opioid effects of BCM7 are questionable since most of BCM7 is degraded during digestion and studies have not established whether or not BCM7 is still present in the bloodstream after someone has consumed milk or casein.[81,82]

It is true that egg and dairy proteins are among the most common food allergy triggers. An estimated 4.7 million adults in the U.S. are allergic to milk, while 2 million U.S. adults are allergic to eggs. (Interestingly, while approximately 10% of U.S. adults have a food allergy, nearly twice as many American adults **believe** that they have a food allergy.[83]) Nevertheless, for those who are allergic to dairy and eggs, they may be able to tolerate dairy products from sheep or goats and only the egg yolk rather than the entire egg (most of the allergenic egg proteins are found in the egg white).

Animal Protein: Muscle's Best Friend

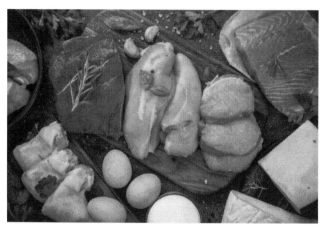

nadianb/shutterstock.com

We talked about the clear superiority of animal protein over plant protein with regard to building and sustaining muscle mass in Chapter 5. Basically, animal protein is more digestible and bioavailable and is ideally equipped with the full gamut of amino acids in the correct proportions that we need for muscle growth and maintenance. Though we've already briefly touched on mTOR (mechanistic target of rapamycin), no discussion of muscle health would be complete without really delving into the subject—mTOR is the major regulator of muscle protein synthesis and muscle mass.

Let's expand upon this all-important signaling hub, particularly as it relates to animal protein.

mTOR

A specific range of mTOR activity is needed for muscle growth and maintenance; too little or too much mTOR activity can result in muscle loss. But before we take a closer look at the connections between muscle, animal protein, and mTOR, I'd like to explain how an imbalance in mTOR activity may be linked to cancer and aging.

Once it's been activated in response to nutrient and environmental inputs, mTOR tells cells to grow and proliferate. Many human cancers are associated with overactivation of mTOR. Since amino acids (from protein) are commonly associated with the activation of mTOR, studies have been conducted to determine whether restricting dietary protein would inhibit cancer growth. Sure enough, observational and animal studies have indicated that a low-protein diet inhibits the growth of various cancers (e.g., prostate, breast), possibly by reducing mTOR activity.[84] Low protein consumption has also been linked to longevity; likewise, inhibition of mTOR in general has been found to extend the lifespan of a variety of species.[85,86]

You're now likely to be totally confused. Reducing dietary protein and mTOR activity runs completely contrary to one of the key tenets of this book, namely that we should eat *more* protein to stimulate mTOR...which in turn would build and maintain our muscles. So what's wrong with this picture? Plenty. Let's dive a little deeper into the complexities of this double-edged sword known as mTOR.

Our bodies maintain a stable internal environment (homeostasis) for many of our internal factors, including our body temperature and blood pressure. That's because any significant deviation from normal levels can have adverse health effects. Similarly, mTOR activity in the body must be balanced. Exercise and high-quality dietary protein cause acute activation of mTOR that drives anabolic processes, i.e., the growth and maintenance of muscle tissue. Conversely, fasting overnight inhibits mTOR signaling so that catabolic processes such as autophagy (recycling, repair, renewal) predominate. Therefore, periodic exercise and normal cycles of eating and fasting *without protein restriction* are sufficient to realize the important health benefits of both high and low mTOR activity. However, prolonged mTOR activity or prolonged mTOR inhibition only leads to bad outcomes. Beyond muscle atrophy, *chronically* activated mTOR from constant eating may promote the development and progression of cancer, other metabolic diseases like diabetes and Alzheimer's disease, and aging.[87] On the flip side, *chronic* inhibition of mTOR from eating a diet low in animal protein can lead to sarcopenia and frailty, particularly in the elderly.[86]

Another key argument against protein restriction centers around inputs other than protein that switch on mTOR, namely insulin and glucose. The increased levels of blood glucose and insulin that occur after meals activate mTOR signaling.[88] *In fact, insulin has been shown to trigger a greater and more sustained activation of mTOR compared with leucine, the primary amino acid that drives mTOR and muscle protein synthesis.*[89] High and frequent consumption of carbohydrates, especially simple sugars, results in the highest blood glucose and insulin levels (compared with protein), and that in turn can lead to chronic mTOR activation. The hyperactivation of mTOR induces cell responses that may lead to metabolic disorders associated with excess carbohydrate consumption, such as obesity, insulin resistance, type 2 diabetes, and non-alcoholic fatty liver disease.[90] The vast majority of snack foods that people consume around the clock—chips, pretzels, crackers, cookies—are carbohydrates and sugars. Accordingly, rather than dietary protein, the *excessive and frequent consumption of carbohydrates* is the real culprit behind the sustained overactivation of mTOR and its associated diseases, along with accelerated aging.

Furthermore, mTOR activity varies between different tissues. Attempting to manipulate mTOR through drastic and unnatural means such as protein restriction may change mTOR signaling in a particular tissue in a way that runs counter to that tissue's preferred level of mTOR activity. Case in point: muscle tissue.

mTOR and Animal Protein

The greater ability of animal protein versus plant protein to stimulate protein synthesis in muscle is due in part to the increased availability of amino acids in animal protein. After an individual consumes animal protein, a rapid and robust rise in essential amino acids appears in the bloodstream, subsequently increasing mTOR activity and muscle protein synthesis. In contrast, consuming plant-based proteins prompts a *lower* rise in amino acids and concurrent *lessening* of mTOR signaling. This was demonstrated in an animal study that compared plant-based proteins (a pea-and-rice vegan mix) with whey protein. Stacked up against the plant proteins, whey produced about a 2-fold larger increase in blood levels of branched-chain amino acids (BCAAs) followed by a 1.5-fold greater increase in mTOR activity. These findings are not unexpected since plant proteins have inferior concentrations of BCAAs, particularly of leucine. Moreover, in a follow-up experiment where plant proteins were fortified to match whey's level of total protein and leucine content, the outcomes did not change—blood amino acid levels and mTOR activity were still higher with the ingestion of whey.[91]

If you still aren't convinced that animal protein is far better than plant protein for the health of your muscles, consider two key points:

(1) As mentioned previously, inhibition of mTOR slows aging and delays the onset of age-related diseases. Eating a plant-based diet is *one way* to lower mTOR.[92] By analogy, some people find that smoking is *one way* to relieve stress and anxiety. Of course, there are healthier ways to reduce mTOR activity (see the next section and Chapter 9) just as there are healthier ways to relieve stress and anxiety. Suffice to say that constant lowering of mTOR via plant-based diets is not conducive to muscle health and in fact increases the risk of sarcopenia and frailty. Shunning superior animal protein is especially detrimental for older adults. As discussed in Chapter 6, anabolic resistance occurs as we age, at which point both exercise *and* protein become less effective at supporting our muscle vitality. So if we assume that maintaining low mTOR signaling via plant-based eating is a healthful strategy, then by extension should we also avoid resistance exercise – a stressor that is a considerably more powerful mTOR trigger than protein??

(2) If plant proteins were superior or even equal in quality to animal proteins, why would companies and researchers be investing time, money, and effort to explore innovative strategies for enhancing the anabolic potential of plant protein?[93]

If you're a vegan, you could just eat more plant protein to compensate for its inferior quality relative to animal protein. Of course, more plant food equals more calories, more carbohydrates, and potentially more weight (fat) gain. *Because consuming protein from plants may be insufficient to maintain muscle health, a strong commitment to regular resistance exercise is critically important for older adult vegans as a way to provide a strong stimulus to muscle.* However, extended periods of inactivity due to injury or illness among vegans (versus among omnivores) may be even more likely to lead to muscle atrophy because of the absence of high-quality, muscle-friendly animal protein in their diets.

Ultimately, with respect to the mTOR story, you have a choice. You can cut back on animal protein in order to possibly live a little longer but run the risk of living out your later years with a frail, weakened body resulting from loss of muscle and bone. Alternatively, you will (hopefully) choose to prioritize animal protein to optimize muscle (and bone) health and likely live just as long or longer, and with a greater likelihood of maintaining functional ability throughout your life.

Minimize Those Carbs

One of the greatest ironies related to our present-day dietary habits is that many people fear eating animal protein but have no concerns about eating endless amounts of processed carbohydrate-based snacks. As you have likely realized by this point in the book, we should be doing the reverse. Recall that maintaining **healthy blood sugar levels** is perhaps the most effective dietary strategy to help prevent diabetes and other major metabolic diseases. In this regard, high protein intake has a favorable effect on stabilizing blood sugar, whereas consuming excess carbs (starches and sugars) increases the likelihood of developing insulin resistance and the consequent elevations in blood sugar levels. Poor blood sugar control caused by eating too many carbs coupled with inactivity is even more likely to occur in those who are already insulin-resistant. That happens to be about *a third of Americans.*

So what about muscle health?

We discussed the potential adverse effects that a high-carbohydrate diet (45% – 65% of calories) has on muscle health in Chapter 4. Basically, compared to a low-carbohydrate diet, a high-carbohydrate diet often leads to a greater loss of muscle mass, and muscle mass is critical for blood sugar control. Meanwhile, swapping proteins for carbohydrates blunts the rise in blood glucose that occurs after meals. Thus, a high-protein/low-carb diet enhances blood sugar control in two ways: directly through blood sugar stabilization and indirectly via its positive effects on muscle health.

To further emphasize this critical point, let's take a look at how a high-carbohydrate diet can undermine muscle health within the context of "chronicity." Chronicity can often be destructive. For example, *acute* inflammation in response to infection or injury contributes to the healing process, but failure to resolve acute inflammation leads to *chronic* inflammation. Over time, chronic inflammation causes the cellular damage that underpins major chronic diseases such as cancer, diabetes, and cardiovascular disease.

In response to a rise in blood glucose, insulin is released in two phases. A rapid and transient "first phase" release of preformed stores of insulin peaks within the first 10 minutes. This is followed by a slowly developing and sustained "second phase" secretion of newly synthesized insulin that plateaus in 2 to 3 hours.[94] The insulin response that results from a diet high in carbohydrates differs from the response that's elicited by a diet high in protein. While both diets generate an early first-phase insulin release, a high-carb diet and *not* a high-protein diet causes a *chronic* release of insulin that remains elevated in the blood 2 hours after eating, driving fat accumulation and inflammation. Moreover, chronic consumption of a high-carb diet produces a strong insulin signal in adipose (fat) tissue but a blunted signal in muscle tissue, resulting in muscle insulin resistance. This effect is reversed when eating a high-protein/low-carb diet.[95] As you may recall, muscle insulin resistance caused by excess carbs contributes to sarcopenia. Excess blood levels of insulin as an early marker of insulin resistance have been associated with the loss of muscle mass in the arms and legs of otherwise healthy older men and women.[96]

Similarly, high levels of insulin and glucose caused by excessive carb consumption induce a chronic activation of mTOR that is accompanied by the health-damaging effects of mTOR being "turned on," so to speak, for too long. Thus, by triggering the chronic activity of both insulin and mTOR, the high consumption of carbohydrates—particularly refined, high-glycemic carbs—contributes to poor muscle health, degenerative diseases, and accelerated aging. On the flip side, individuals who challenge themselves *intermittently* with exercise and fasting (see the next chapter) can to some degree counteract the *chronicity* of mTOR and insulin activity that results from a high-carbohydrate diet. The payoff is low insulin levels and balanced mTOR signaling, which prompts body fat to be burned for fuel *and* which maintains optimal muscle mass and strength.

But let's go beyond the molecular biology and biochemistry and view the carbohydrate dilemma through an evolutionary lens by asking a basic question: what is the major difference between our ancient hunter-gatherer diet and our modern Western diet? (Common sense also comes into play here.) Our ancestors ate animals, fish, vegetables, fruits, nuts, seeds, and occasional tubers. Today, we eat those same foods...BUT with the addition of a myriad of processed carbohydrate-rich foods: bread, pasta, rice, potatoes, pancakes, waffles, bagels, crackers, pretzels, etc. *Could all of those carbs be the real culprit behind today's epidemic of degenerative diseases? Could the lack of those carbs be why we also lacked those diseases in our ancient past?*

My answer to both of those questions is a resounding "Yes!" I maintain that it's (almost) all about the insulin. Directly as well as indirectly through its negative influence on muscle health, chronically elevated insulin that results from excess carbs, the wrong fats (trans fats such as margarine, excess omega-6 fats from seed oils, fats that have oxidized after being subjected to high heat), and sedentary living is tightly linked to today's scourge of metabolic diseases, from diabetes and obesity to cancer and Alzheimer's disease. Chronically elevated insulin is also what's behind the increasing incidences of sarcopenia and osteoporosis.

Since our bodies have a small, limited supply of stored carbohydrate, reliance on carbohydrate foods as our primary fuel leads us to constantly eat in order to maintain our energy levels and avoid extreme hunger. As you may recall from Chapter 2, around 75% of adults are carbohydrate-intolerant. For these people, eating too many carbs becomes a liability—they are far better off limiting their carbs. But even for those 25% or so who can tolerate moderate to high amounts of carbs without adverse health effects, the aging process will likely flip the script seeing as carbohydrate intolerance increases with age. Moreover, most people don't actually know whether or not their genetic makeup will allow them to thrive on a higher-carb diet for the long term. That's why the far safer bet is to *up the protein and lower the carbs.*

All things considered, if we want optimal muscle health, it would seem prudent to keep our consumption of carbohydrates on the low to moderate side (25% – 40% of our total calories) rather than at the higher government-recommended levels (45% – 65% of calories). (See Chapter 11 for how these percentages translate into actual food portions.) Not only is low to moderate carbohydrate consumption better for muscle maintenance, it's also associated with decreased risks for obesity, metabolic syndrome, type 2 diabetes, and cardiovascular disease.[97] Eating more than half of our calories as carbohydrates provides no health benefits—it only causes potential problems.

If you're truly ambitious, give keto a try! Reducing carbs to ketogenic levels, particularly when combined with intermittent fasting, will cause insulin levels to plummet. While keto is not easy and is not for everyone, its health benefits are truly remarkable! More about that next.

The Modified Ketogenic Diet: The Flip Side of High-Carb

The ketogenic diet takes carbohydrate consumption to another level. To be more specific, the hallmark of the ketogenic diet is a very low intake of carbohydrates: only 5% – 10% of total calories. Most people need to restrict carbohydrate consumption to less than 50 grams/day in order to maintain a state of nutritional ketosis, i.e., elevated blood ketones. However, people vary widely in terms of how much they need to restrict carbohydrates in order to trigger ketogenesis (formation of ketones). Some people can achieve nutritional ketosis with 100 grams of carbs per day, while others need to drop down to 20 grams of carbs per day.[98]

Nutritional ketosis is a natural metabolic state that develops when dietary carbohydrates are limited or unavailable. Once carb intake drops low enough to suppress insulin and deplete liver glycogen, the liver converts body fat and dietary fat to water-soluble ketone bodies, or ketones. Thus, instead of carbs, fats and their ketone byproducts become the body's primary fuel sources. Beta-hydroxybutyrate (BHB) is the predominant ketone in the body; nutritional ketosis occurs when there's between 0.5 and 3.0 mmol of BHB in the blood.[99]

While the essential feature of the ketogenic diet is very low carb intake, an optimal protein intake of around 20% – 35% of calories is absolutely critical. This amount should be based on the amount of protein intake needed to support muscle health (see Chapter 5). While some people may need to eat less protein to achieve ketosis, *it is far more important to eat enough protein to support muscle mass.* Unlike the traditional ketogenic diet, this "modified" keto diet puts a premium on dietary protein over ketones. Individuals may use other measures such as fasting and/or consuming medium-chain triglyceride (MCT) oil to generate more ketones to compensate for the reduced ketone production from higher dietary protein (which can convert to sugar) that some people experience.

Fat consumption comprises the remaining calories and should be maintained at a level needed to support either a stable weight or weight loss. If you're pursuing a modified keto diet, you should get about 60% – 80% of your total calories from fat, and that fat should be comprised primarily of saturated and monounsaturated fats, *not* seed oils. Unless you have hypertension and are being medically treated, you should also consume about 4 – 5 grams/day of extra sodium by salting foods and/or consuming broth or bouillon. Also eat plenty of potassium-rich foods such as avocadoes and non-starchy veggies and consider a magnesium supplement, particularly if you're experiencing muscle cramps.

Overwhelming evidence suggests that dietary saturated fat does not pose a risk to your health. It is the high consumption of carbs rather than saturated fats that raises *blood levels* of saturated fats. Once your body becomes adapted to a low carbohydrate intake (particularly the level that qualifies as a very low "keto" level), you'll preferentially burn off saturated fat for energy rather than glucose. That means that (due to low insulin levels) saturated fat won't be deposited in your fat tissues. *In order to optimize your use of fat and ketones as dominant fuels, you'll need to adapt to a very low-carbohydrate diet. This is paramount. Know that it can take up to 6 weeks to become fully adapted.*[98]

Keto Preserves Muscle

Contrary to the widely believed notion that restricting carbohydrates leads to muscle loss, the low-carb ketogenic diet actually has quite the opposite effect. Nutritional ketosis induced by the keto diet exerts an anti-catabolic effect. In other words, muscle mass is preserved because muscle protein is not broken down for energy use.[100] This is evidenced by a study that compared three diets with equal amounts of calories and protein but differing amounts of carbohydrate. The diet with the fewest carbs (30 grams/day) caused an increase in ketones and resulted in more fat loss than the other diets did. More importantly, lean tissue (muscle) was preserved to the greatest extent on the keto diet.[101] Thus, the utilization of protein is improved during nutritional ketosis. This may allow you to eat less protein on keto while still maintaining your muscle mass. *However, more protein (30 to 50 grams per meal) is always better, as in a modified high-protein keto diet. Due to anabolic resistance, this is particularly important for older adults!*

Mechanisms

One potential mechanism whereby the ketogenic diet preserves muscle during aging relates to the alliance between muscles and nerves. Muscle function relies on the nervous system to transmit signals to muscles in order to trigger the contraction and relaxation of muscle fibers. The loss of nerve supply to muscle fibers is a hallmark of various types of muscle loss, including sarcopenia. The ketogenic diet may potentially reverse this age-related "denervation" atrophy of muscle.[102]

In a study in mice, a long-term ketogenic diet was shown to mitigate sarcopenia partly through "reinnervation," i.e., restoring nerve function to muscle (see illustration below). In addition, the keto diet resulted in greater numbers of mitochondria and antioxidants, which may have led to the preferential preservation of oxidative muscle fibers over glycolytic fibers. In plain English, the keto diet shifted fuel utilization toward fat, which can be burned by oxidative muscle fibers. Glycolytic muscle fibers, in contrast, rely on the burning of glycogen for energy. These adaptations may have fostered a healthier cellular environment—namely, less oxidative stress and inflammation—that led to the reduced formation of abnormal (unfolded) proteins, thus lessening the need for protein synthesis to replace any deformed or damaged proteins. As a result, with less protein turnover, muscle mass and function were better maintained even in the midst of advancing age.[102]

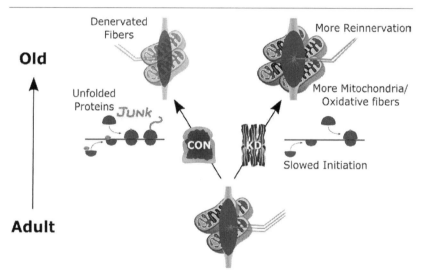

Reprinted with permission from Wallace M.A., Aguirre N.W., Marcotte G.R., Marshall A.G., Baehr L.M., Hughes D.C., Hamilton K.L., Roberts M.N., Lopez-Dominguez J.A., Miller B.F., et al. The ketogenic diet preserves skeletal muscle with aging in mice. Aging Cell. 2021;20:e13322.

As muscle progresses from adult to old, mice on a standard control diet (CON) show less reinnervation and more unfolded (abnormal) proteins. By contrast, mice on a long-term keto diet (KD) showed more mitochondria, greater reinnervation, more oxidative muscle fibers, and decreased protein synthesis (slowed initiation). This resulted in significantly greater muscle mass with aging among the KD mice compared to the CON mice.

Another potential mechanism of the keto diet involves the conservation of branched-chain amino acids (BCAAs). Among the essential amino acids, BCAAs (particularly leucine) are the most effective at not only triggering muscle growth but suppressing muscle breakdown as well. In another special role, BCAAs can serve as a major direct source of energy for muscle cells during exercise.

Blood levels of BCAAs are significantly increased on the keto diet. Because ketones and BCAAs are structurally similar, during ketosis, ketones may be preferentially burned for energy, thus sparing BCCAs for muscle maintenance.[100] Intravenous infusion of the ketone beta-hydroxybutyrate in volunteers resulted in a decreased use of leucine for energy—instead, protein synthesis was enhanced.[103]

Lastly, a "protein-boosting" effect has been seen with supplemental ketones. Recall that a special protein called mTOR is a major player in building muscle mass. When taken after exercise, BHB markedly enhanced the mTOR signaling stimulated by leucine. This increase in mTOR activity led to a doubling of protein synthesis.[104]

Evidence

A limited number of human studies have investigated the ability of a low-carbohydrate ketogenic diet to support gains in muscle mass with resistance training. In a recent study in college-aged athletes, the anabolic effects of the keto diet were compared with a traditional Western diet having identical calories and protein. Following 10 weeks of resistance training, gains in muscle mass and reductions in body fat in the keto group matched the gains in the traditional group.[105] In another study, keto-induced muscle gains *without the inclusion of a structured resistance exercise program* were surprisingly observed. A 6-week carbohydrate-restricted diet resulted in a significant but unexpected increase in lean body mass (along with decreased body fat) in a group of healthy, normal-weight men. These men transitioned from a diet of 48% carbs to a keto diet of 8% carbs.[106]

While other studies examining resistance exercise on the keto diet did not show similar muscle gains, they at least demonstrated muscle preservation. In one such study, elite gymnasts followed a keto diet for 30 days, during which they performed their normal training program. This resulted in a substantial decrease of their body fat and fat percentage without compromising their strength or power performance. Muscle mass was basically maintained (though there was a nonsignificant increase).[107] Similarly, in a study of non-elite CrossFit athletes, the keto diet induced major losses in body fat while preserving muscle mass. CrossFit is a high-intensity training program that incorporates weightlifting and other resistance exercises. All of the participants in the study significantly improved their total CrossFit performance time and overall power.[108]

Beyond Muscle

The health benefits of ketosis are so wide-ranging that it sounds almost too good to be true! Yet research continues to accumulate that supports the diverse applications of ketosis, from improved endurance athletic performance to the treatment of epilepsy and cancer. What's particularly noteworthy, a meta-analysis published in 2021 in the journal *Nutrition Reviews* found that the ketogenic diet was superior to control diets at controlling blood sugar and reducing body weight for up to 6 months in people with obesity and type 2 diabetes. Improvements in blood levels of triglycerides and HDL particles—as well as reduced use of anti-diabetic medications—continued for up to 12 months for those on the keto diet.[109]

When they're in the state of ketosis, people often report having sharper mental focus, better appetite control, increased fat loss, and of course improved body composition. What more could you want? Well, here's another perk: higher levels of ketones can help you maximize your muscle. Think of the keto diet as a powerful tool in your nutritional toolbox that can be utilized periodically or continuously for its tremendous muscle and health benefits. Once again, *you need sufficient time—up to 6 weeks—to become adapted to a keto diet and develop the necessary metabolic flexibility to burn both fat and carbohydrates.* This adaptation period is critical to people's success with a ketogenic diet.

That said, for many people, a low to moderate carb intake may be sufficient to promote optimal muscle health. The choice depends on individual health and fitness goals as well as inherent needs and weaknesses. While the keto diet is generally not very appealing to carb devotees, there are still plenty of tasty alternative ingredients readily available (such as nut flours and other non-grain-based flours) that can make the diet suitable for those who absolutely cannot be deprived of breads and bread products.

Chapter 9

Intermittent Fasting

The idea that fasting can help preserve and regenerate muscle seems counterintuitive. How can avoidance of food, particularly protein, benefit muscle health? In short, fasting activates autophagy, a little-known "housekeeping" mechanism that plays an essential role in muscle maintenance. But before we elaborate on how fasting benefits muscle health, let's examine the nuts and bolts of the increasingly popular practice of intermittent fasting.

The emergence of intermittent fasting in recent years may appear to be a novel approach to improving health. However, it's not unprecedented! Involuntary fasting (periods of famine) is entrenched in human evolution, while voluntary fasting for religious or therapeutic reasons has been practiced for thousands of years. Today, backed by abundant evidence from animal and clinical studies showing that fasting provides tremendous health and longevity benefits,[1,2] the popularity of intermittent fasting (IF) is very much on the rise. I believe every health improvement book should include a section on IF for the express reason that *eating less often is one of the greatest drivers of longevity!*

Simply stated, IF entails taking periodic breaks from eating. For recurring periods of 12 hours up to potentially several days, all calorie-containing foods and beverages are prohibited or highly restricted. A brief description of the various types of IF is summarized below[3]:

Different Methods of Intermittent Fasting

Time-Restricted Feeding (TRF)	Eating within narrow time windows (typically 4 – 12 hours) while fasting for periods of 12 – 20 hours on a daily basis.
Alternate-Day Fasting (ADF)	Alternating calorie-free fasting days with feast days of unlimited consumption of food and beverages.
Alternate-Day Modified Fasting (ADMF)	"Fasting" days consisting of consuming fewer than 25% of daily calorie needs are alternated with feast days of *ad libitum* (liberal) food and beverage consumption.
Periodic Fasting (PF)	Calorie-free or very-low-calorie fasting periods are cycled for consecutive days ranging from 2 to as many as 21 or more days.

Time-restricted feeding (TRF) is one of the most popular and well-tolerated IF methods, particularly the 16:8 or 18:6 versions that involve fasting for 16 or 18 hours and eating for 8 or 6 hours. This deviates significantly from the typical eating window of about 15 hours as well as from the notorious "round-the-clock" eating pattern. Skipping breakfast is the easiest strategy for TRF (if you miss having breakfast foods, simply eat them at lunch or dinner), though some people may prefer to skip dinner. Simply delaying breakfast and/or eating an early dinner can work as well. On the whole, TRF is the "easiest" and safest way to fast. I do it daily, and highly recommend it.

Some studies have indicated that late-night eating (dinner immediately before bed or snacks after dinner) is linked to poor health.[4,5] On the other hand, other research data suggest that consuming about 30 – 40 grams of pre-sleep protein (particularly slow-release casein protein) about 1 – 3 hours prior to sleeping may contribute to overall muscle enhancement.[6] While the jury is still out with regard to eating close to bedtime, the key to IF is to allow for a sufficient gap without calories. That's a gap of about 12 – 20 hours, preferably a gap of at least 16 hours.

Among the wide-ranging health benefits linked to IF are weight (fat) loss, lower heart rate and blood pressure, reduced inflammation, and—in particular—increased insulin sensitivity. Owing in part to the improvement in insulin sensitivity, IF has been shown to protect against and even reverse type 2 diabetes. *(Note: medical supervision is imperative for people with diabetes who wish to fast.)* Growing evidence also suggests that IF may contribute to the prevention and treatment of major chronic disorders such as obesity, cardiovascular disease, cancer, autoimmune disease, and neurodegenerative diseases (e.g., Alzheimer's disease and Parkinson's disease). Last but not least, like calorie restriction, IF has been shown to increase lifespan in a wide variety of species.[7,8]

So how does this age-old practice of fasting confer such impressive benefits? For the most part, fasting mediates these effects through a phenomenon called "hormesis." Hormesis is a process whereby a mild "good" stress—a short-term lack of food, exercising, or getting mild sun exposure—elicits an adaptive beneficial response that increases resilience against more formidable future stressors and promotes resistance to disease. Because exercise and fasting represent forms of adversity, they are also referred to as "adversity mimics." To quote the German philosopher Friedrich Nietzsche, "What does not kill me makes me stronger."[9]

Intermittent fasting induces adaptive responses by cells via the following cellular and molecular mechanisms[2,10]:

(1) Reduced oxidative stress
(2) Decreased inflammation

(3) More efficient mitochondrial energy metabolism

(4) Enhanced repair and elimination of damaged molecules and organelles (autophagy)

The central driver of the remarkable health benefits of IF—the one that intersects with each of the four underlying mechanisms—is the *intermittent* flipping of a "metabolic switch" that shifts the body's primary energy source from glucose to fats and fat-derived ketones.[11] This shift in fuel preference is prompted by the depletion of liver glycogen (the body's storage form of carbohydrate) and is regulated primarily by hormonal signaling from low insulin levels. Liver glycogen is depleted after 12 to 36 hours of fasting, depending upon the quantity of glycogen stored in the liver prior to the fast as well as the amount of energy expended (exercise) during the fast. It is no coincidence that the recommended TRF fasting windows of at least 16 and up to 20 hours are in keeping with this timespan (usually beyond 12 hours) required for liver glycogen exhaustion and the flipping of the metabolic switch.

When the metabolic switch is turned "on" during fasting, the creation of new mitochondria and improved mitochondrial function (fueled by ketones and fatty acids) enables more efficient energy production that's needed for cell protection, repair, and survival. This adaptive response to fasting (i.e., greater numbers of better-functioning mitochondria) persists beyond the fast to promote disease resistance. (Conversely, mitochondrial *dysfunction* contributes to chronic diseases.) During refeeding when the switch is "off," growth, proliferation, and remodeling predominate.

The fasting-induced transitioning of metabolic fuels from glucose to fat and ketones leads to greater metabolic flexibility. Such flexibility was a survival advantage for our hunter-gatherer ancestors, enabling them to store fat when food was abundant and utilize fat as a fuel when food was in short supply. This inconstancy of the food supply (which was the original form of intermittent fasting) was the rule for the vast majority of human existence.[12] In today's world, however, an abundance of food and our frequent consumption of high-glycemic snack foods precludes periods of fasting. This leads to an inability to access and burn fat and ketones for energy—in other words, metabolic *inf*lexibility—and the consequent accumulation of body fat.

Importantly, in contrast with the *chronicity* of a calorie-restricted diet, *intermittency* (switching back and forth between consuming calories and not consuming any) is the key feature of fasting. Intermittency is what imparts the distinct benefits of IF, namely enhanced cellular rejuvenation and stem cell activation. These benefits are associated with the refeeding or "recovery" phase, which of course is absent in continuous calorie restriction.[8] It's similar to exercising—during the *recovery* period after exercise is when the "magic" happens in the form of increased muscle size and strength.

Intermittent fasting may be contraindicated for select groups of people, including children, breastfeeding and pregnant women, underweight or malnourished individuals, and the elderly. In addition, fasting may not be appropriate for people with immunodeficiencies (e.g., those on medical immunosuppressants), eating disorders, traumatic brain injuries, or dementia.[13] Interestingly, animal studies have suggested that fasting may be beneficial when patients are fighting bacterial infections but harmful when patients are challenged by viral infections; hence the adage "Feed a cold, starve a fever."[14]

Health Benefits of Fasting

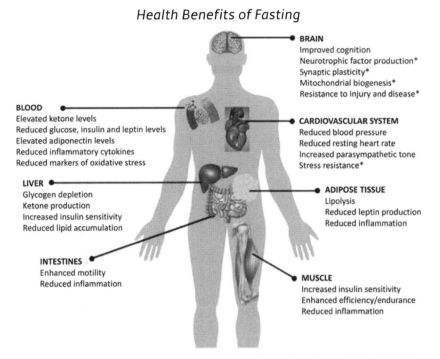

BRAIN
Improved cognition
Neurotrophic factor production*
Synaptic plasticity*
Mitochondrial biogenesis*
Resistance to injury and disease*

BLOOD
Elevated ketone levels
Reduced glucose, insulin and leptin levels
Elevated adiponectin levels
Reduced inflammatory cytokines
Reduced markers of oxidative stress

CARDIOVASCULAR SYSTEM
Reduced blood pressure
Reduced resting heart rate
Increased parasympathetic tone
Stress resistance*

LIVER
Glycogen depletion
Ketone production
Increased insulin sensitivity
Reduced lipid accumulation

ADIPOSE TISSUE
Lipolysis
Reduced leptin production
Reduced inflammation

INTESTINES
Enhanced motility
Reduced inflammation

MUSCLE
Increased insulin sensitivity
Enhanced efficiency/endurance
Reduced inflammation

Source: Reprinted with permission from Anton, S.D., et al., Flipping the Metabolic Switch: Understanding and Applying the Health Benefits of Fasting. Obesity (Silver Spring), 2018. 26(2): p. 254-268.

Intermittent Fasting and Muscle Health

Unlike doing resistance training and eating more animal protein, people don't usually fast for the sole purpose of supporting and enhancing their muscle health. Most people who fast are doing it for other reasons, such as weight management, blood sugar control, and overall health improvement. Since weight reduction is often at the top of the list for many practitioners of fasting, it's reassuring to know that weight loss from doing short-term IF (e.g., TRF, ADF) mostly comes from losing body fat—lean muscle mass is spared.[11] However, lifestyle interventions work best when practiced in concert. For example, increases in muscle fiber size are driven by the synergistic effects of resistance training and dietary protein. By the same token, the preservation of muscle tissue during IF may be compromised if an individual's dietary protein is subpar and/or they are not exercising. But here's more good news: the retention of lean mass during IF has been shown to be improved by both endurance and resistance exercises.[15,16]

A study published in 2020 in the *Journal of the American Medical Association* (JAMA) claims that much of the weight loss from intermittent fasting and specifically time-restricted feeding comes from muscle.[17] Does this finding suggest that IF is harmful to muscle health? Quite the contrary! This study clearly underscores how critical it is to *also* eat sufficient amounts of dietary protein and exercise while fasting in order to maintain muscle health. Study participants were *not* instructed to alter their diet in any way or make any changes to their physical activity. Changes in protein intake were *not* measured; as noted by the authors, this may have accounted for the loss of lean mass. It is certainly plausible that by skipping breakfast, the participants' daily protein intake was reduced. To make up for lost calories, they may have eaten more high-carb convenience foods, something that's certainly not conducive to maximizing muscle health. And in addition to eating less dietary protein, reduced physical activity may have also contributed to the loss in their lean mass—the daily step count decreased significantly for the people in the fasting group compared to the control group.

Similarly, a negative impact on lean mass was also observed in a TRF study in which protein intake was intentionally decreased by 30 grams/day.[18] However, no changes in lean mass were observed in a follow-up study in which protein intake did not differ from pre-study consumption.[15]

According to a review of studies by leading authorities on IF, an estimated one-fourth to one-third of weight loss resulting from continuous calorie restriction is lean mass.[11] In contrast, when compared to a normal control diet, TRF matched for protein intake was found to decrease body fat and maintain muscle mass in resistance-trained males.[15] Moreover, in calorie-restricted diets, a protein intake of 1.2 grams per kilogram of body weight (which is higher than what the RDA suggests) had a stronger sparing effect on muscle mass and was shown to be necessary for preserving participants' resting metabolic rate, thus lowering the risk of weight regain for the dieters.[19] This finding would likely apply to IF as well since people who practice IF regimens usually end up eating fewer calories (though not intentionally).

How Fasting Spares Muscle

One mechanism by which IF preserves muscle mass is through autophagy—fasting is a particularly potent activator of the body's natural quality control and recycling process.[20] Autophagy plays an essential role in muscle integrity and performance. Numerous studies have shown that autophagy preserves muscle and strengthens muscle fibers through the regeneration of new fibers from stem cells. However, uncontrolled or defective autophagy accelerates muscle atrophy.[21] (See Chapter 6 for a more in-depth discussion of autophagy and its role in muscle health.)

Another mechanism connected to the sparing of muscle during fasting involves the shift in energy metabolism from burning glucose to burning primarily fat and ketones in muscle mitochondria. Damaged or dysfunctional muscle mitochondria are major contributors to muscle loss, particularly as we age.[22] Since fat and ketones are "cleaner"-burning fuels compared to glucose, fewer mitochondrial free radicals are generated that would otherwise damage mitochondria. In addition, fasting drives the creation of new mitochondria (mitochondrial biogenesis) as well as the destruction and elimination of defective mitochondria in muscle cells.[11] Thus, fasting restores balance and quality to the mitochondrial pool in muscle, with the overall effect of more efficient energy creation and—very importantly!—muscle preservation.

The retention of muscle protein during fasting is also driven by growth hormone (GH). Fasting enhances the overall secretion of GH by increasing the frequency and strength of distinct periodic GH pulses (bursts). Increased GH secretion during conditions of stress (e.g., fasting and exercise) has been preserved throughout human evolution to spare our muscle protein and ensure our survival.[23] This muscle-conserving effect of GH is mediated in muscle directly by GH itself and indirectly through the synthesis and release of another anabolic hormone: insulin-like growth factor 1, or IGF-1. Research suggests that the mechanism of action of growth hormone appears to be mostly the suppression of muscle protein breakdown rather than the synthesis of muscle protein— experimentally suppressing GH during fasting has been shown to *increase* muscle protein breakdown by about 50%. This is another indirect effect of growth hormone prompted by its stimulation of the breakdown of fats to release fatty acids and generate ketones which are preferentially used as fuels, thus sparing the use of muscle protein for energy.[24]

Lastly, given that every cell contains protein, the first proteins that are broken down for glucose during fasting are those that turn over most rapidly, such as gut and skin cells. Muscle cells, in contrast, turn over less often and are thus largely preserved.

A closing note on this topic: if you find fasting to be too challenging, try going on a ketogenic diet for a few weeks. Like fasting, following a keto diet will enable you to flip your metabolic switch and burn fat (and ketones) more readily for energy, thus avoiding carb/sugar cravings and dips in your blood sugar. This may make it easier to transition to fasting.

Chapter 10

Evidence-Based Supplements

There's certainly no shortage of nutritional supplements claiming to improve exercise performance! However, the alleged performance-enhancing properties are unsubstantiated for the vast majority of such products. Nevertheless, there are several evidence-based nutritional products that can complement the ability of resistance exercise to increase muscle protein synthesis (MPS) and/or suppress muscle protein breakdown (MPB) to achieve a positive muscle protein balance and help resist the age-related loss of muscle mass. These nutritional supplements include protein (e.g., whey), branched-chain amino acids/leucine, vitamin D, omega-3 fatty acids, creatine, MCT oil, carnosine, L-carnitine, collagen peptides, HMB (beta-hydroxy-beta-methyl butyrate), and glutamine.

Whey Protein

While consuming sufficient dietary protein is critical for muscle maintenance, supplemental protein (typically in the form of protein powders) is not essential. That said, there are several compelling advantages to using supplemental protein, particularly when coupled with resistance training. Among supplemental proteins, whey protein is superior for supporting muscle mass and health.[1] Since it's also the most commonly used protein supplement to support muscle gains, we're going to focus on whey protein.

Whey is the liquid byproduct of the production of cheese and yogurt. It accounts for 20% of the protein in cow's milk, with casein making up the majority (80%). However, whey protein is a more potent stimulus of MPS than casein (and soy). Data from many studies suggest that the whey fraction of milk is what drives milk's exceptional ability to promote muscle growth and strength gains following a bout of resistance exercise.[1]

The greater MPS response from whey is due its unique makeup. Being an animal-derived protein, whey is a complete protein of the highest quality, which is to say that it contains all of the essential amino acids (EAAs) *in the proper balance*. It's especially rich in a group of EAAs called branched-chain amino acids (BCAAs)— leucine, isoleucine, and valine—that play an important role in tissue growth and repair. Leucine in particular is a key catalyst for MPS via its independent activation of mTOR, the master regulator of MPS. Whey has a high proportion of leucine, registering at about 12%. (In contrast, grain proteins only have about 6% leucine.[2]) Furthermore, whey is quickly digested and absorbed into the bloodstream, resulting in a rapid and marked rise in blood levels of leucine and other amino acids. This accelerated elevation of blood leucine levels is vital for the optimal stimulation of MPS.[1]

As discussed in Chapter 5, whey protein is second to none as a post-exercise recovery food. Whey protein speeds recovery from muscle damage caused by intense exercise. In a study of 24 healthy young men, compared with a placebo supplement, supplementation with whey protein was shown to accelerate the increase in satellite cells (muscle stem cells) induced by high-intensity exercise.[3] Muscle satellite cells are vital for muscle health and function, particularly muscle regeneration, turnover, and growth. This increase in satellite cells was largely associated with type II muscle fibers. As you may recall, type II fibers are engaged by *intense exercise* and are more prone to age-related atrophy than type I fibers are.

Many active people are already rewarding themselves with tasty whey shakes after strenuous workouts. Beyond workout recovery, whey protein can be leveraged for additional important benefits, including upgrading the quality of your overall protein intake. In a study of healthy older adults, consuming whey protein without changing total calories was shown to partly offset some of the adverse effects of short-term physical inactivity from bed rest. Compared with a control group on a mixed diet, subjects who consumed whey protein lost about 50% less lean mass and had a greater loss of body fat. Notably, following rehabilitation, diminished muscle strength in the whey group fully recovered, while diminished strength persisted in the control group.[4]

Consistent with the findings reported here thus far, whey protein can help optimize body composition by promoting and maintaining weight (and fat) loss. This effect may be mediated through appetite suppression. For example, in a study of lean, healthy men, a whey protein meal produced an effect superior to other protein meals (e.g., tuna, turkey, eggs) in significantly reducing hunger and increasing fullness while also reducing *ad libitum* (liberal) food intake at a subsequent meal.[5] A meta-analysis of 14 randomized controlled trials confirmed that whey protein combined with resistance exercise significantly decreases body weight and body fat while increasing lean body mass.[6]

Furthermore, whey protein can help control blood sugar levels, thus contributing to improved weight management and a lower risk of diabetes. Consuming whey protein may be a simple and inexpensive way to lower blood sugar surges that would otherwise occur after meals. In a randomized clinical trial of people with well-controlled type 2 diabetes, consuming whey protein shortly before eating a breakfast of high-glycemic-index foods increased insulin secretion and reduced after-meal blood glucose levels by 28%.[7] This *transient* rise in insulin induced by whey protein is in stark contrast to the *sustained* elevation in insulin levels (reflected in high fasting insulin) that is caused by persistent high blood sugar and insulin resistance. Chronically elevated insulin circulating in the blood—not short-lived bumps—is what increases the risk of obesity and age-related degenerative diseases.[8] Indeed, in overweight/obese individuals, whey protein has been shown to improve insulin sensitivity, thus minimizing the amount of insulin these individuals need to lower their blood sugar.[9] Once again, this transient insulin spike induced by whey protein is another example of the benefits of *intermittency* (much like IF and intense exercise) versus the negative effects of *chronicity*.

Exercise aside, drinking a whey protein shake is a convenient way to ensure sufficient protein intake when practicing time-restricted feeding (see Chapter 9). When following an 18:6 or 16:8 eating schedule, it just isn't practical to fit three major meals into a 6- or 8-hour window. Eating two meals and a light snack is a more workable schedule. If you wish to maximize your muscle and minimize your body fat, drinking a delicious whey protein beverage in lieu of a light snack can significantly boost your total daily protein intake while minimizing your total calories.

Branched-Chain Amino Acids/Leucine

As previously noted, the muscle-enhancing effects of whey protein are primarily mediated by its high concentration of the branched-chain amino acids (BCAAs): valine, isoleucine, and particularly leucine. BCAAs represent nearly half of the essential amino acids in food and 35% of the total amount of essential amino acids that construct muscle proteins.[10] Among the BCAAs, leucine is the most important as it alone can trigger muscle protein synthesis, even when an individual is at rest. However, recent evidence suggests that supplementation with *all* of the BCAAs after resistance exercise stimulates MPS more potently than supplementation with leucine alone.[11] More notably, neither BCCAs as a whole nor a standalone leucine supplement are capable of *maximizing* and sustaining the MPS response following resistance exercise without the presence of a complete protein source (such as whey protein).[12,13] In other words, a full complement of essential amino acids as contained in a complete protein food is required for maximal MPS that is sustained for 2 – 3 hours after exercise. In fact, supplementation with either BCAAs or just leucine after resistance training does not impart significant additional benefits to a workout recovery beverage that contains a sufficient amount of whey protein (i.e., 20 – 40 grams).

On the other hand, supplementation with BCAAs and/ or leucine may be more appropriately utilized as a means of bolstering a suboptimal dose of a complete protein to achieve a greater anabolic effect. For example, adding a high dose of leucine to a beverage containing a small amount of whey protein (6.25 grams) was demonstrated to stimulate MPS to the same extent and duration as four times as much whey protein alone (25 grams). While the addition of BCAAs to the low-protein beverage also increased MPS, it was less effective than both the supplemental leucine plus 6.25 grams of whey protein and the higher 25-gram dose of whey protein alone.[14]

Older adults *require* more dietary protein but *consume* less protein than younger adults. Several factors account for the progressive decline in protein consumption as people age, including diminished appetite, increased and prolonged satiety, impaired chewing capabilities, changing food preferences, lower calorie needs, and economic and cultural barriers. Leucine supplementation may provide important muscle benefits in older adults. The satiating effects of a larger meal (more protein) for older individuals may be eased by substituting that with a smaller meal (less protein) supplemented with leucine, all while still increasing MPS to support muscle mass. Considering that protein consumption is generally mixed with other macronutrients (carbs and fats) that may effectively lower an individual's ability to absorb amino acids, it has been suggested that older adults should consume a higher leucine dose of 4.5 grams or more per meal.[15] This would necessitate supplementing suboptimal protein meals with about 3 grams of leucine to overcome the blunted MPS response of muscle (i.e., anabolic resistance) that's common in older persons, thus counteracting the development of sarcopenia.[16]

Though not as potent as standalone leucine in fortifying suboptimal protein meals, supplemental BCAAs may nevertheless aid in muscle recovery after resistance exercise. Conversely, leucine alone has been reported to be comparatively ineffective within this context.[17] Muscle damage caused by intense exercise triggers an acute inflammatory response wherein injured cells are cleared by specialized immune cells called "macrophages."[18] This pro-inflammatory phase is followed by a prolonged restorative phase in which inflammation is resolved and muscle is regenerated. Blood levels of creatine kinase or CK—a biomarker of exercise-induced muscle damage—increase during the late regenerative phase of tissue injury. Two systematic reviews with meta-analyses of randomized controlled trials demonstrated that BCAA supplementation can potentially reduce muscle damage and muscle soreness in trained males after resistance exercise. Notably, the release of CK into the blood was reduced, suggesting a specific role for BCAAs in accelerating exercise recovery by activating muscle regeneration.[19,20]

So how do these findings relate to muscle function and physical performance?

Muscle damage from resistance training is associated with a parallel decline (5% – 7%) in power-producing ability, such as jump height, muscular strength, and submaximal endurance performance. In a study in resistance-trained males, supplementation with 20 grams of BCAAs in a split dose prior to and following an intensive strength-training session significantly counteracted the training-induced decreases in power-producing ability compared to placebo ingestion.[21] (This was assessed by measuring the performance of countermovement jumps and seated shot-put throws.)

Beyond their ability to trigger muscle growth and accelerate post-exercise recovery, branched-chain amino acids can be burned directly in muscle cells as an energy source to fuel prolonged exercise when carbohydrate stores become depleted. Supplementation with BCAAs prevents fatigue during endurance events partly by lowering the concentration of serotonin, a central fatigue substance.[22] Cyclists and marathoners have reported reduced times when using BCAAs immediately before and during events. In a placebo-controlled study published in 2021 in the *Journal of Science and Medicine in Sport*, 18 recreationally active men undergoing a prolonged cycling time trial experienced significantly improved performance and reduced ratings of perceived exertion while ingesting BCAAs.[23]

Creatine

Creatine is a compound made up of three amino acids: methionine, arginine, and glycine. Stored primarily in muscle tissue (about 95%), creatine derives its name from the Greek *kreas*, meaning "meat."[24] About half of the daily requirement of creatine is naturally synthesized in the body while the other half is obtained largely from seafood, meat, and poultry. (Vegan diets are not only low in creatine but its precursor amino acids as well.) Creatine is one of the most popular and well-documented sports supplements for increasing muscle mass, strength, and power in both younger and older adults, particularly when combined with resistance training.[25,26]

The central metabolic role of creatine is to link with phosphorus to form phosphocreatine, an energy molecule that's stored in muscle cells. Phosphocreatine reversibly transfers a high-energy phosphate molecule to ADP (adenosine diphosphate) to regenerate ATP (adenosine triphosphate), the energy currency of the cell. Phosphocreatine is utilized during exercises such as weightlifting and sprinting that require brief, all-out exertion lasting up to around 6 seconds. Most of the stored phosphocreatine is depleted within 10 seconds of the onset of exercise, resulting in rapid muscle fatigue. Evidence suggests that saturating muscle cells with supplemental creatine will conserve ATP and hold back fatigue, thus enhancing athletic performance in sports involving high-intensity, short-duration efforts (especially in those who eat little meat).[27,28] Moreover, when paired with resistance training, creatine supplementation leads to a roughly 3-pound greater increase in lean tissue mass (compared with a placebo), accompanied by significantly greater increases in upper and lower body strength.[29]

Beyond athletics, creatine may support muscle mass and function in older adults, particularly in those who are creatine-deficient or at high risk of deficiency (e.g., those with reduced appetites, vegetarians, and vegans). A review of studies concluded that even without resistance training, creatine supplementation may counteract the age-related loss of muscle mass and muscle strength at least partly through its ability to restore energy depletion. Some of these studies suggest that creatine may also suppress inflammation, increase bone strength, and reduce the risk of falls.[26] Furthermore, seeing as it has also been shown to improve memory and cognition, creatine may even play a role in preventing and treating neurodegenerative diseases such as Alzheimer's disease and Parkinson's disease as well as strokes.[25]

Typically, the whole-body pool of creatine in someone weighing about 150 pounds is 120 grams, with 2 grams per day obtained from both the diet and the body's natural production of creatine. While creatine supplementation causes a reduction in endogenous (self-made) synthesis, this is reversible when supplementation is discontinued.[25] A dosing strategy of 3 grams per day of creatine monohydrate—the most popular form of creatine—for 28 days will result in muscle saturation of creatine. By comparison, eating about 1 ounce of dry beef daily without including any other dietary source of creatine means that it will take an individual about 240 days to achieve saturation of creatine in their muscle. Supplementation of 3 grams of creatine a day can be continued long-term. Another effective approach is loading on about 5 grams of creatine monohydrate four times per day for 5 – 7 days followed by a maintenance dosage of 3 – 5 grams/day.[15] Short- and long-term creatine supplementation (up to 30 grams per day) is safe and well tolerated and does not appear to adversely affect liver or kidney function in older adults.[30]

Omega-3 Fatty Acids (EPA & DHA)

Oily fish are our main dietary source of EPA (eicosapentaenoic acid) and DHA (docosahexaenoic acid), the most biologically active omega-3 fatty acids. Evidence continues to accumulate that demonstrates the benefits from dietary supplementation with fish oil rich in EPA/DHA for a wide range of chronic diseases, including type 2 diabetes, metabolic syndrome, cancer,

Alzheimer's, and particularly various cardiovascular diseases.[31-33] The greater an individual's consumption of EPA/DHA is from food or supplements, the lower their risk is of dying from any cause.[34]

While the main claim to fame of omega-3 fatty acids is supporting the health of our heart muscle, these remarkably versatile nutrients appear to benefit our skeletal muscle as well. When ingested, omega-3 fatty acids are appreciably incorporated into the membranes of our muscle cells, resulting in pronounced effects on muscle metabolic and physical function.[35] EPA and DHA appear to enhance the sensitivity of muscle to anabolic triggers (e.g., resistance exercise, protein ingestion, and insulin) and to increase the activation of mTOR, the master regulator of muscle protein synthesis. Studies in adults of all ages have demonstrated that daily supplementation with a moderate dose of about 4 grams of EPA/DHA increased mTOR signaling and enhanced the increase in MPS response to a constant infusion of amino acids and insulin.[36,37]

The anabolic effects of omega-3 fatty acids may be

Fish Oil Storage and Alternative

Unlike stable saturated fats such as butter, the omega-3 polyunsaturated fats found in fish oil are unstable and very susceptible to oxidation (rancidity) from exposure to light and heat. Therefore, fish oil pills should always be stored in an opaque container and be tightly resealed after having been opened. Also, ALWAYS REFRIGERATE FISH OIL! Purchase fish oil from a reputable company like Nordic Naturals or Life Extension and be sure that antioxidants such as vitamin E have been added to it. If you cannot tolerate fish oil, consider krill oil as an alternative and follow same storage precautions. The omega-3 fats in krill oil are actually more bioavailable than omega-3s derived from fish oil and are particularly beneficial for brain and joint health. Ideally, choose a product with omega-3 fats from both fish and krill sources as they complement each other.

especially beneficial for older adults. The ability of exercise to prevent and reverse sarcopenia is well-established. However, exercise adaptations—including improvements in muscle mass and strength, greater numbers of muscle satellite (stem) cells, and the creation of new energy-producing mitochondria—are blunted in older adults. This anabolic resistance to strength training (as well as to protein) is in large part responsible for sarcopenia, the age-related loss of muscle mass and strength that leads to diminished physical function and future disability. In healthy older adults, daily supplementation with about 4 grams of EPA/DHA for 16 weeks increased muscle protein synthesis before and after a single bout of resistance exercise.[38] A study in elderly women showed that fish oil supplementation enhanced their neuromuscular response to strength training, resulting in greater improvements in muscle strength and functional capacity.[39] Moreover, *even without resistance exercise*, daily supplementation of omega-3 fatty acids for 6 months in healthy older adults has been shown to increase muscle mass and strength.[40] All in all, these studies support the ability of omega-3 fatty acids to enhance anabolic responses to exercise as a means to combat anabolic resistance and protect against sarcopenia in older adults.

Apart from aging, periods of physical inactivity (e.g., bed rest) hasten the progression of anabolic resistance and sarcopenia. Omega-3 fatty acid supplementation may be an effective intervention to counteract the muscle atrophy that occurs after intervals of muscle disuse. In a study of 20 healthy young women, participants had one of their legs immobilized in a set position for 2 weeks followed by 2 weeks of return to normal activity. Supplementation with 5 grams/day of EPA/DHA or sunflower oil (control) was initiated 4 weeks prior to immobilization. Omega-3 supplementation was found to mitigate the decline in muscle size and mass associated with 2 weeks of muscle disuse. Moreover, muscle bulk fully recovered to pre-immobilization levels in the omega-3 group only.[41]

Vitamin D

While its classical function is to facilitate normal bone mineralization, vitamin D is associated with approximately 800 human genes that govern many critical functions in the body. There has been an explosion of research in recent years linking low levels of vitamin D to many chronic diseases, including cardiovascular disease, cancer, diabetes, Alzheimer's disease, and autoimmune disorders. That being the case, it should not be surprising to know that vitamin D also plays a critical role in muscle health and function and that its shortage may increase the risk of sarcopenia.[15]

Through the activation of the vitamin D receptor, vitamin D supplementation in *people with low serum levels* triggers muscle protein synthesis followed by an increase in the size and number of type II muscle fibers, which in turn leads to greater muscle strength.[42] In support of these findings, treatment of cultured muscle stem cells with vitamin D or its active form resulted in increases in muscle fiber size, including a significant 2-fold increase in the mean diameter of the fibers and a 2.5-fold increase in their length.[43,44] Vitamin D is also implicated in muscle damage repair and regeneration. In a randomized, placebo-controlled trial in 20 vitamin-D-deficient males, supplementation with a generous dose of vitamin D3 (4,000 IU/day) elevated serum vitamin D levels and significantly improved functional recovery from damaging eccentric (muscle-lengthening) contractions of the knee extensors at 48 hours and at 7 days after the exercise. In contrast, no changes in the recovery rate were observed in a placebo control group.[45]

Worldwide, low vitamin D levels are a major public health concern. Older adults are particularly at an increased risk of vitamin D deficiency due to a number of factors, including poor intestinal absorption and limited sun exposure. A greater decline in physical performance and an increased risk of limited mobility and disability in elderly individuals are associated with serum vitamin D levels below 20 ng/ml (normal serum vitamin D levels are 30 – 100 ng/ml).[15] A systematic review and meta-analysis found a synergistic effect from combined vitamin D supplementation (400 – 2,000 IU/day) *and* resistance training for the improvement of muscle strength in older adults; however, any evidence of this benefit from vitamin D supplementation alone was lacking.[46]

Interestingly, according to another review of studies, higher doses of vitamin D3 appear to have ergogenic (performance-enhancing) potential through increased aerobic capacity, muscle growth, force and power production, and shorter recovery time from exercise. Researchers determined that dosages of vitamin D3 ranging from 4,000 – 5,000 IU/day together with 50 – 1,000 mcg/day of a mixture of vitamins K1 and K2 are vital to health and maximal athletic performance.[47] (Vitamins K1 and K2 prevent arterial calcification and vitamin D toxicity.)

Carnosine

Found exclusively in animal tissue, carnosine is a nonessential dipeptide molecule that consists of two amino acids: beta-alanine and L-histidine. While it is synthesized in the body, carnosine can also be obtained from the diet, mostly from meat and fish. (Similar to creatine, carnosine was named after *carnis,* the Latin word for "meat."[48]) Carnosine is capable of exerting strong antioxidant, anti-inflammatory, and anti-glycation effects in the body. Accordingly, studies suggest that carnosine supplementation may play a role in the prevention of chronic diseases such as type 2 diabetes, cardiovascular disease, and neurodegenerative diseases, as well as aging in general.[49] Nevertheless, the preponderance of evidence for carnosine supplementation pertains to improved exercise performance.[48,49]

The vast majority of carnosine is concentrated in muscle. Since type II (fast-twitch) muscle fibers contain 30% – 100% more carnosine than type I (slow-twitch) fibers do, people whose muscle is made up of predominantly type II fibers will have comparatively greater concentrations of muscle carnosine.[50] Recall from Chapter 7 that type II muscle fibers are more prone to atrophy than type I fibers are. Thus, in older adults, a lack of intense exercise needed to maintain type II muscle fibers contributes to loss of both muscle and carnosine with advancing age. Supplementation with L-carnosine at dosages of 1,000 mg/day and 2,000 mg/day has been shown to significantly increase muscle carnosine content.[51] High muscle carnosine content improves exercise performance, particularly high-intensity exercises lasting from 1 – 4 minutes.[48] In older adults, increased muscle carnosine is associated with improved exercise tolerance and delayed fatigue.[49]

The ergogenic effects mediated by carnosine appear to be primarily due to an increase in the buffering capacity of muscle. Carnosine increases the ability of muscle to buffer excess acid (acidosis) in the blood that results from high-intensity exercise. Acidosis is a major contributing factor to the onset of muscle fatigue. Other possible mechanisms of action for carnosine include suppression of oxidative stress and improved exercise capacity.[48]

MCT Oil (Medium-Chain Triglycerides)

MCT oil is a concentrated source of medium-chain triglycerides (MCTs). This oil is becoming increasingly popular as an energy-boosting and fat-burning supplement. MCT oil is extracted primarily from coconut oil and derives its unique benefits from its smaller size—whereas most dietary fats are long-chain triglycerides (LCTs) containing 12 carbons, MCTs are only 6 – 12 carbon links long (hence its name of "medium-chain"). The smaller size of MCTs allows them to be easily absorbed and rapidly converted to energy in the liver. In fact, these fats are burned for energy as quickly as glucose is!

MCTs can also swiftly generate ketones (ketone bodies). Caprylic (C8) acid and capric (C10) acid are the specific MCTs in the oil that drive the production of ketones, which is an alternative fuel source for the muscle, heart, and brain cells. While the anti-obesity and anti-diabetic effects of MCTs are well-established, emerging evidence supports a role for MCTs in protein metabolism as well as in muscle strength and function.

Hunan and animal studies suggest that MCTs are effective for improving muscle health even under unhealthy conditions. In a three-month randomized controlled trial, supplementation with 3 grams/day of MCTs in frail elderly adults significantly improved major measurements of muscle strength and function (e.g., hand grip strength, knee extension time, walking speed) compared with supplementation of equal amounts of LCTs.[52] Previous to this study, the same researchers had observed similar positive results with the combined supplementation of MCTs, leucine, and vitamin D.[53] Consumption of MCTs may also prevent muscle atrophy induced by inactivity. In rats fed an MCT-enriched diet followed by leg immobilization, atrophy of the soleus muscle in the calf was partially suppressed, whereas muscle mass in the soleus of rats fed an LCT-enriched diet markedly decreased.[54]

Muscle atrophy can be caused by an imbalance between the rates of muscle protein synthesis and muscle protein degradation. Inactivity-induced muscle atrophy in particular appears to primarily involve an increase in protein degradation independent of a decrease in protein synthesis (the latter may not always occur).

Research evidence suggests that at least some of the protective effects of MCTs on muscle wasting are mediated by the inhibition of immobilization-induced increases in the production of a specific enzyme (MuRF-1) that tags and destroys various proteins in the body, including the myofibrillar proteins that make up muscle fibers. More precisely, the suppression of excessive muscle fiber degradation by MCTs appears to be facilitated by beta-hydroxybutyrate, a MCT-derived ketone body.[54]

While research supporting the direct benefits of MCTs to muscle health is limited, the ketones generated from MCTs may be the principal driving force behind their favorable effects on muscle and overall health. As discussed in Chapter 8, high-energy ketones spare muscle from being degraded to its constituent amino acids for the creation of new glucose (gluconeogenesis). Ketones also enhance the signaling of mTOR, the master regulator of muscle protein synthesis. Finally, due to their similar structures, ketones are preferentially burned for energy to spare the essential branched-chain amino acids—including the all-important leucine—for the building and repair of muscle tissue. (Otherwise, the BCAAs would be used for muscle energy demands.)

Glutamine

Glutamine is the most abundant free amino acid in the human body, with a high concentration found in muscle cells. It has multiple metabolic functions, including energy production, ammonia detoxification, glycogen synthesis, and the regulation of protein synthesis and degradation. It's a nonessential amino acid because it's synthesized in the body from other amino acids. However, during stressful conditions involving tissue damage (e.g., illness, trauma, burns, intense exercise) the body's own production of glutamine, primarily in muscle, may not be adequate and additional glutamine must be obtained from foods or supplements. Thus, glutamine is considered to be a *conditionally essential* amino acid.

Because exercise and particularly resistance training is a significant stress that damages muscle, supplemental glutamine may exert its greatest benefit in muscle recovery from exercise. In a randomized controlled study consisting of 16 healthy volunteers, glutamine supplementation after knee extension exercise resulted in significantly faster recovery as demonstrated by reduced strength loss and muscle soreness compared with a placebo. The ability of glutamine to suppress inflammation and promote muscle protein synthesis may account for these muscle recovery effects.[55] In a study of exercising elderly women, 30 days of glutamine supplementation at 10 grams/day improved the strength and power of the participants' knee muscles as well as their blood sugar control and antioxidant status. The latter metabolic benefits may be due to enhanced insulin signaling in muscle and higher levels of glutathione, the body's master antioxidant.[56]

L-Carnitine

Like creatine and carnosine, L-carnitine is found almost exclusively in animal foods (red meat being the richest source) and likewise has a name that signifies meat—carnitine is derived from *carnus*, the Latin word for "flesh." It is not an essential nutrient since it is also synthesized in the body (from the amino acids lysine and methionine). L-carnitine plays an essential role in energy metabolism by transporting fatty acids to the mitochondria, where they are burned for energy. For this reason, L-carnitine is highly concentrated in skeletal muscles and the heart—tissues that primarily burn fats for fuel.[57]

L-carnitine supplementation may improve exercise performance and recovery. In a study of resistance-trained athletes, supplementation with 2 grams/day of L-carnitine for 9 weeks improved upper and lower body strength as reflected in significant increases the number of reps and sets on the bench press and the leg press. A considerable increase in anaerobic power during the Wingate test (a 30-second cycle test) was also observed, as well as significant reductions in blood lactate and markers of post-exercise inflammation and oxidative stress, both of which indicated an enhancement of the recovery process.[58]

Apart from its ergogenic effects, L-carnitine may improve muscle health in older adults. The amount of L-carnitine stored in muscle declines with age in healthy people. Evidence from a review of studies suggests that L-carnitine can increase muscle mass in older people and restore their age-related decline in muscle functioning. We may be able to infer a possible mechanism for this from an animal study showing that the ability of L-carnitine to convert fat into energy allows branched-chain amino acids to be spared for muscle protein synthesis rather than be burned for energy.[59]

HMB (Beta-Hydroxy-Beta-Methylbutyrate)

HMB (beta-hydroxy-beta-methylbutyrate) is a byproduct formed from the breakdown of the branched-chain amino acid leucine. Human and laboratory studies have shown that HMB triggers muscle protein synthesis and curbs muscle protein breakdown.[60] Athletes have been using HMB supplements for years to increase muscle mass, strength, and endurance. However, the scientific evidence for HMB's muscle-enhancing effects is suspect as more recent clinical trials and reviews have suggested little or no effect. Nevertheless, HMB may be useful for preventing muscle atrophy associated with inactivity and aging (though again, evidence for this is limited).

HMB supplementation of 3 grams twice daily over 6 months was shown to improve strength, body composition, functionality and muscle quality in both sedentary and resistance-trained adults who were aged 65 years and older.[61] In another study in older adults, HMB supplementation prevented muscle loss during 10 days of bed rest and promoted gains in leg muscle mass and strength after an 8-week exercise rehabilitation program.[62] While both HMB and leucine reduce muscle loss in older adults, HMB may have a more favorable effect due its more prolonged action—it has a longer half-life in the blood. Moreover, the conversion of leucine to HMB has been reported to be reduced by 25% in adults aged 65 years and older.[63] Beyond muscle health, some evidence suggests that HMB can also potentially be used to reduce abdominal obesity and improve bone density and cognitive function in older adults.[64]

Collagen Peptides

Collagen peptides (a.k.a. hydrolyzed collagen) are dietary supplements produced by the enzymatic hydrolysis of food proteins. During this process, collagen extracted from animal sources is broken down into small protein fragments called "peptides." This hydrolyzed collagen is water-soluble and thus more easily digested and more rapidly absorbed. Studies have shown that ingested collagen peptides are detected in the bloodstream and can effectively stimulate the synthesis of collagen in the body.[65]

Recent studies in both healthy adults and elderly men with sarcopenia have reported that collagen peptide supplementation in combination with resistance training can significantly increase muscle strength and fat-free mass (includes muscle, bone, water, organs, and connective tissues).[65-68] However, researchers were unable to determine whether *muscle* was the tissue affected by collagen peptides since muscle protein synthesis was not measured in these studies. Other researchers did in fact measure rates of MPS and showed that collagen peptides paired with RT in healthy older women did not significantly increase MPS above baseline levels. High-quality whey protein was found to be more effective at supporting muscle preservation, thus slowing age-related muscle loss.[69] Moreover, collagen is a low-quality protein—it's low in essential amino acids, particularly leucine. (Remember, leucine is the primary trigger for both mTOR and increased rates of MPS.) Leucine concentrations in collagen peptides are only 0.4 grams per 15 grams of collagen, far below the 3 grams of leucine needed to stimulate MPS.[66]

On the other hand, some studies have shown that the nonessential amino acids glycine and proline (which are highly concentrated in collagen) may play a role in muscle enhancement. In animal models, glycine has been shown to activate mTOR and protect against muscle wasting.[70] Also, a collagen dipeptide consisting of the amino acids hydroxyproline (a derivative of proline) and glycine was shown to promote the growth of cultured muscle cells from mice via the mTOR pathway.[71]

Another explanation for the increase in fat-free mass from collagen peptides may be related to their ability to drive collagen synthesis, as previously stated. It's plausible that rather than acting on muscle cells per se, collagen peptides increase the collagen content of the structural connective tissue distributed around the muscle cells.[68] Also recall that hydroxyproline—which is abundant in animal foods but scarce in plants—is a key constituent of collagen and has been demonstrated to significantly improve the health of bones and joints (connective tissue and cartilage) as well as skin and the intestines.[24]

Chapter 11

Putting It All Together

Now it's time to put everything you've learned in the preceding chapters into action! As you do so, you'll optimize your physical functioning, protect against chronic diseases, and add more healthy years to your life. And you'll do all of these things within the context of muscle health. Greater muscle mass is independently associated with longer and better-quality survival among older adults. Conversely, a decline in muscle mass can potentially lead to debilitating frailty, impaired metabolic health, and accelerated aging. For individuals in that situation, the last years of their lives can be quite harsh.

The good news is that muscle loss and bodily deterioration as we age are *not* inevitable! Professional athletes and bodybuilders who continue training throughout their lives (though to a lesser degree in retirement) maintain most of their robust muscularity. They are living proof that muscle mass can be preserved throughout life. But athletes aside, anyone can push back on age-related muscle loss. By following the recommendations in this book, *you can rebuild your muscle and maintain it.* It is never too late to implement these lifestyle strategies to preserve your precious muscle and maintain your independence throughout your life. ***It is imperative that you hold on to your muscle as you grow older!***

Regular exercise is essential. Exercise, *particularly the intense variety*, restores a more youthful expression of genes that control aging. *We evolved to exercise; we were built to move.* While any exercise is good, resistance training is the key to muscle maintenance and should be an integral part of everyone's exercise regimen. Increasing your muscle mass and strength will put less demand on your cardiovascular system because there will then be fewer (though individually stronger) muscle fibers it has to support when you need to perform a particular activity. Conversely, muscle loss and a weaker body will put more strain on your heart and vascular system since those systems will need to service a greater number of weaker muscle fibers required to complete a specified task. In essence, resistance training both preserves your muscle *and* improves your cardiovascukar fitness.

With regard to diet, the prevailing belief is illogical and misleading—although we are told that eating more plant foods and fewer animal foods will put us on the path to improved health, nothing could be further from the scientific truth. Yes, plant foods contribute fiber and important antioxidant nutrients and polyphenol pigments to our diet. However, we humans are far more carnivorous than herbivorous. Animal foods give us the most concentrated and *bioavailable* assortment of muscle-enhancing nutrients on the planet! And these foods do *not* cause disease or death. (See Chapter 8 for more info on why.) Furthermore, with its high percentage of carbs, the American diet is *already* plant-based and has been for decades, ever since the "fear of fat" came into play in the 1980s. The outcome of pursuing this plant-based—one could say plant-*biased*—diet is an alarmingly high number of American adults who today are metabolically *un*healthy.

That said, don't skimp on nutritious non-starchy veggies and moderate amounts of low-sugar fruits! But *prioritize* animal protein by eating *at least* 4 – 6 ounces of high-quality, easy-to-digest animal protein three times a day. These are the foods (meat, fish, eggs, full-fat dairy) that we're literally made of! These animal-sourced foods will make you thrive, not just survive. Rather than deteriorate, your muscles (and bones) will prosper.

Speaking of eating, take a break now and then. Constantly eating does not allow your body to repair damage and clean up cellular debris. In contrast, the simple practice of restricting your eating window to 6 – 8 hours to allow for a 16- to 18-hour-long fast does wonders for your muscle – including better muscle definition - and overall health. Intermittent fasting is a quality-control mechanism that preserves muscle mass by degrading damaged proteins and promoting the differentiation of muscle stem cells into fresh new muscle fibers. *Eating less often is one of the most important lifestyle change you can make to live healthier and longer!*

Lastly, try viewing your lifestyle through an evolutionary lens. Most hunter-gatherer societies subsisted on a diet high in animal proteins/fats and low in carbohydrates. They certainly endured periods of famine and were unlikely to be eating three square meals a day. Needless to say, their levels of daily physical activity (particularly intense activity) were off the charts. These *intermittent* adversity mimics—intense exercise and fasting—were the norm. Importantly, this high-protein, low-carbohydrate diet as well as periodic food shortages and high levels of physical activity were programmed into our human genome over thousands of years. Perhaps we should look to our distant ancestors for lifestyle clues. After all, they endured harsh environments, yet remained largely free of the chronic diseases of civilization (obesity, diabetes, heart disease) even when they reached an advanced age.

So let's put it all together:

1) **Do some *intense* exercise***
   Exercise should be a priority for everyone in the same way that eating and sleeping need to be priorities. Any exercise is better than no exercise. However, intense exercise is

a game changer! Exercising at intensity levels above the lactate threshold (i.e., being winded or training to the extent of muscle failure or fatigue) causes lactate levels in the blood to increase substantially. This was once considered a liability, a concept that many people still wrongly believe. To the contrary, high lactate levels in the blood stimulate the release of a cascade of hormones (among them, growth hormone) and other substances that underlie many of the body's adaptations to exercise that rejuvenate muscle and overall health, including cardiorespiratory fitness and metabolic health. *High-intensity exercise is also the best exercise you can do to activate your longevity genes.* What's not to like?!

Be consistent! Even on days when you cannot perform your normal routine, just get out of breath. That's the secret! For example, do some sit-ups or push-ups until you are winded. Remarkably, your body will respond to this very brief but intense adversity (low oxygen and energy) by boosting your resilience and activating your anti-aging genes.

- **Resistance training**

  Top priority should be given to resistance training (RT), which is pushing or pulling against resistance. The resistive load can be free weights (dumbbells and barbells), weight machines, elastic bands, medicine balls, your own body weight, or anything that causes muscle contraction. RT can be performed 2 – 3 nonconsecutive days per week, with a dose of 2 – 4 sets of 8 – 12 repetitions per muscle group. However, even a single session per week may suffice depending on your intensity of effort. The greater the workout intensity, the longer the recovery, and the fewer sessions needed.

Five simple compound exercises that hit all of the major muscle groups may be all you need as a solid foundation. These exercises include the chest press, seated row, lat pulldown, overhead press machine, and leg press. The free-weight equivalent to machines includes the barbell row, overhead barbell/dumbbell press, dead lift, bench press, and squat. Importantly, *RT should be performed to muscle failure (fatigue).* That's the point at which another repetition is not possible.

Amazingly, even doing RT for 3 seconds a day (e.g., a single bicep curl) performed 5 days a week over a period of 4 weeks has been shown to increase muscle strength! Once again, the "secret sauce" was *maximal effort*—working to the point of muscle fatigue.

- **High-intensity interval training**

  High-intensity interval (HIIT) workouts involve short, intermittent bursts of vigorous exercise interspersed with recovery periods of rest or lower-intensity exercise. HIIT is bittersweet—it's demanding but brief. Any exercise mode (e.g., cycling, walking, swimming) can be adapted for HIIT workouts. Consider using a cardio machine such as the elliptical trainer.

  Typically, a high-intensity interval workout consists of intense effort for 5 seconds – 8 minutes at 80% – 90% of maximal heart rate (submaximal). These short bouts of exercise are separated by 1 – 3 minutes of recovery at low intensity or by complete rest. A single workout session of alternating exercise and recovery continues for 3 – 4 cycles (totaling 20 – 60 minutes) and performed 2 – 3 times per week. For beginners, a simple approach is to break up a walk or jog with 3 – 4 all-out sprints of 50 – 100 meters, sufficiently spaced out.

A more demanding version of HIIT is sprint interval training. SIT is characterized by a 30-second all-out (supramaximal) effort followed by a longer recovery of 4 – 5 minutes. With warm-up and cool-down, 4 cycles of SIT can be completed in 25 minutes, but only 2 minutes of those cycles are intense. As SIT is extremely strenuous, it is more appropriate for athletes and physically fit people.

- **No better duo of high-intensity exercises**
  It would be hard to beat the duo of RT and HIIT! Pairing resistance training with high-intensity interval training will provide you with the ultimate partnering of intense exercise for muscle health and general health as well as longevity.

- **Exercise while fasting**
  Ideally and if your schedule permits, exercise (especially the intense variety) while fasting. Doubling down on these adversity mimics will give you greater health benefits—including muscle enhancement and intensified fat burning—than either challenge alone. If this isn't feasible, try to at least double down once or twice a week. Do your intense workouts while fasting on weekends, for example, or whenever your schedule allows. You will still reap superior benefits.

  Think of your first meal as a deserving reward for having put your body through adversity twice over. Follow the feast and famine model—it's programmed into our human genome! *Intermittent* (not chronic) adversity triggers survival mechanisms that promote longevity.

- **Work out at your own pace and take time to recover**
  The amount of high-intensity exercise each of us needs is extremely variable. It depends on a person's age, goals, current health and fitness status, and the level of exercise

intensity performed. *The key is to allow adequate recovery time between sessions.* Start slow and increase your intensity and frequency gradually. You may start off with one resistance training session per week and add a second session as you get stronger. Intersperse RT with one or two sessions of HIIT workouts. Avoid back-to-back HIIT sessions. On days when you're not doing intense workouts, you may rest, walk, or engage in activities of low to moderate intensity (e.g., yoga, Pilates).

Set the bar high! Challenge yourself periodically—every now and then, try lifting more weight or sprinting faster or walking a longer distance. If you fail to improve but you break even, you've won! Instead of regressing, you're maintaining. You're beating aging.

Once again, the greater the intensity, the longer the recovery. Even if you require 7 days of recovery, you will still realize significant muscle and health benefits. Progress according to how your body feels. It's trial and error. *Do not overtrain.*

*My intent here is not to provide detailed exercise protocols but to suggest the basic types of exercise that are best for optimal muscle health. Many of you will be workout veterans and well ahead of the game. If you are new to exercise, however, consider seeking out a trainer to get started. And if you have a health issue, always consult your doctor before embarking on an exercise program.

2) **Prioritize high-quality proteins**
   - **Eat 30 – 50 grams of high-quality protein three times per day.**
     Make it easy by tracking your protein intake on a meal-to-meal basis. Ideally, aim for 30 – 50 grams (4 – 6 ounces) of high-quality protein at each of your

Animal Protein Sources

Meat that is 100% grass-fed is preferred over conventional feedlot meat because it's more environmentally friendly and has a better nutrition profile. However, it may be difficult and/or expensive to always consume grass-fed meat. Moreover, the nutritional differences can easily be compensated for by other foods—oily fish provides far more omega-3 fats than grass-fed beef does. Most importantly, both types of meat will stimulate muscle. On the other hand, poultry and eggs should always be pastured (these are typically easier to find and less expensive), dairy should be naturally full-fat, and fish should be from sustainable, wild-caught sources (such as wild Alaskan salmon and other sustainable wild fish; check out seafoodwatch.org for more information). In any case, PRIORITY should always be given to high-quality protein over consuming more carbs. This is paramount!

three meals regardless of your body size. This meal threshold of 30 grams of protein provides the roughly 3 grams of leucine you need to fully stimulate your mTOR. (Remember, that's the master regulator of muscle protein synthesis.) *Ideally, eat about 40 grams or more of protein during your first and last meals, when muscle protein synthesis is most favorable.* This will trigger a big anabolic effect and will serve as the lion's share of your total daily protein needs (again, make it simple and shoot for about 1 gram per pound of body weight per day). Your midday meal should still provide at least 30 grams of protein in order to support stable blood sugar levels, regulate your appetite, and amp up your metabolism.

Because I strongly recommend time-restricted eating, it may be challenging to eat three meals within a 6- to 8-hour period. Therefore, when you're not exercising, you can substitute a quickly digested, leucine-rich whey protein beverage for a full meal to round out your total daily protein allotment. If you'll be drinking the whey shake *after* exercising, read the following sections closely to maximize your protein.

- **Choose animal proteins**

  Animal proteins (meats, fish, eggs, full-fat dairy) are high-quality and clearly superior to lower-quality plant proteins with regard to muscle protein synthesis and the maintenance of muscle mass. Eat 4 – 6 ounces of any meat, fish, eggs, or dairy (full-fat cheese or yogurt) three times a day. Nothing complicated here. As a rule of thumb, 1 ounce of meat/fish/cheese provides about 7 grams of protein, an egg gives you 6 grams, and a cup of full-fat milk or whole-milk yogurt gives you 8 grams of protein. See sample menus for ideas about how to incorporate these foods into your daily diet.

- **Include collagen-rich foods**

  Though it is a lower-quality protein, collagen is nevertheless an important structural protein found in connective tissues such as cartilage, bones, tendons, ligaments, and skin. And it's even critical for the structure and function of skeletal muscles. Good dietary sources of collagen include bone broths, the skins of poultry and fish, sardines, and organ meats, e.g., liver, tripe, heart, brain, sweetbreads, and kidneys. Shoot for 3 – 4 servings per month. *However, do not substitute these foods for high-quality animal proteins (excepting sardines).*

- **Consume whey protein after exercising**

  Exercise sensitizes muscle to the anabolic effects of protein, so during the post-exercise recovery period, it's best to consume 20 – 40 grams of protein to maximize muscle protein synthesis. Ideally, drink a whey protein shake *without carbs*, preferably within 2 hours of your workout. If you're an older adult, shoot for 40 grams, particularly if this is your first "meal" of the day. Tip: drink down your whey beverage in short order rather than sip on it leisurely.

3) **Minimize carbohydrates**

Carbohydrates are like interior car accessories—they make driving more comfortable and convenient, but your car will run just fine without them. It would likely run even better! Some of those accessories—dash-mounted TV screens, in-car microwaves, window tinting—can even be risky. Too many can be quite costly.

Such is the case with dietary carbohydrates, or more precisely, starches and some sweet fruits. Let's call these "glycemic carbs" because they spike your blood sugar. Unlike fats and proteins, our bodies do not require *dietary* carbohydrates. (The exceptions to this are athletes who rely on carbs for energy and are not adapted to a ketogenic diet.) Thus, dietary carbs are optional. How many carbs you eat daily is your personal choice. Of course, *do* eat plenty of non-starchy veggies and moderate amounts of low-sugar fruits (see Appendix), but for *most* people, the overwhelming evidence suggests keeping glycemic carb consumption to a minimum.

Eating refined, processed carbs and sugars is akin to pouring gasoline onto a fire. A high-glycemic carbohydrate intake is not consistent with our hunter-gatherer past and typically undermines protein nutrition, which is critical for optimizing muscle health. On top of that, an excessive intake of glycemic carbs is likely a major factor in the current epidemics of obesity and diabetes, both of which are linked to insulin resistance. And remember, insulin resistance contributes to age-related muscle loss.

- **Low-carbohydrate diet**

  For optimal muscle health, keep carbohydrate intake on the low to moderate side (25% – 40% of your total calories), favoring the lower end. At 25% of calories, an 1,800-calorie meal plan would provide about 112 grams of carbohydrates in the form of, for example, 1 sweet potato, 1 apple, 6 servings of non-starchy veggies, 1 cup of blueberries, and 1 cup of full-fat Greek yogurt. Again, keep things simple. Every day, think about eating only one starch, a couple of low-sugar fruits, and plenty of non-starchy veggies. Choose low-glycemic carbs such as unprocessed whole-grain products and whole fruits over quick-digesting high glycemic carbs such as refined grain- and sugar-based products. (Note that fruit juices are very sugary.)

- **Very-low-carbohydrate diet (ketogenic)**

  A more challenging though highly rewarding option is to restrict carbohydrate consumption down to a range of 20 – 50 grams per day. This very low carb intake will usually trigger the generation of ketones and will keep an individual in a state of nutritional ketosis. High levels of ketones in the body are associated with remarkable health benefits, including increased muscle protein synthesis and the preservation of muscle mass. Unless you have hypertension and are on medications, be sure to consume extra sodium to the tune of 4 – 5 grams/day (consider consuming 1 – 2 cups of broth or bouillon daily). Eat high-potassium foods such as avocados and non-starchy veggies. You may want to consider a magnesium supplement if you experience muscle cramps or fatigue.

If you wish to try the keto diet, I suggest a 30-day trial in order to become keto-adapted. Being "keto-adapted" means that your body has learned to optimize its use of ketones and fats as its dominant fuels. Ideally, cut out all starches and eat 1 – 2 daily servings of fresh low-sugar fruits such as berries, melons, or peaches. A serving of full-fat yogurt can be worked in as well. You don't need to eat enormous amounts of fat—the key to keto is slashing your carbs intake. Of course, as always, ***prioritize animal protein!***

After a 30-day trial, you can stay the course or cycle in some carbs 1 – 2 days per week while still remaining in ketosis (high blood ketones). These "carb-loading" days should still be on the low side, i.e., 25% – 40% of your total calories. You may find that you perform high-intensity exercise better on carb-loading days.

There are endless options for modifying a keto diet while maintaining ketosis. For example, high-intensity exercise, fasting, and MCT oil can all elevate blood ketone levels and may be used to compensate for "cheating" with added carbs. On the other hand, carbing up on weekends to high levels (45% – 65% of calories) will likely thwart many of the benefits of keto regardless of taking these additional measures.

- **No one-size-fits-all approach**

  All in all, a low to moderate carb intake may be sufficient to promote optimal muscle health provided that you put a premium on animal protein. On the other hand, you may opt for the more aggressive keto approach or just use the keto diet periodically as a powerful tool in your nutritional "toolbox." Along with contributing to enhanced muscle health, very low carb consumption will cause your fasting insulin to nosedive, thus bolstering your insulin sensitivity and significantly reducing your risk of metabolic disease, e.g., obesity, type 2 diabetes, cancer, and heart disease. It appears that each individual's degree of underlying insulin resistance is a major factor that determines that person's appropriate amount of carb consumption. My recommendation is simple: **keep your carb intake low, at around 25% of your total calories**. However, if you can tolerate keto (or close to it), go for it!

Keep Omega-3 and Omega-6 Fats in Balance

A high ratio of omega-6 to omega-3 fats—the two main types of essential polyunsaturated fats—drives muscle-damaging inflammation. We evolved eating a diet with an omega-6 to omega-3 ratio of 1:1 to 3:1, but our typical grain-based Western diet today features a whopping ratio of 20:1! This huge shift in the types of fat we consume has largely been due to the emergence of industrial RBD seed oils (refined, bleached, and deodorized) like corn, canola, and soy oils as well as countless processed foods that contain RBD oils and trans fats. The solution? Replace highly processed foods with non-starchy veggies and eat two or more servings of oily fish per week (and/or supplement with 2 – 4 grams of fish oil).

Nothing beats it. You will likely attain your best results, especially with regard to body composition (a.k.a. you will be shredded!). Remember, as you adapt to burning ketones and fats for fuel, it gets easier and easier to maintain that status. *But always keep starches and sugars low!*

4) **Don't obsess over dietary fat**

   In the context of a low-carbohydrate diet, fat is not the enemy provided that you eat the right types. Choose saturated fats (from meat and dairy) and monounsaturated fats (from olive oil, avocado, nuts, and, yes, beef!) for energy in lieu of carbs. Eat grass-fed butter and full-fat cheeses and yogurt. There's no need to trim the fat off meat or avoid the skin of poultry...after all, skin is rich in collagen! Avoid/limit highly polyunsaturated oils such as corn oil and soybean oil as they are more susceptible to oxidation (rancidity) and potentially promote tumor growth. (In contrast, saturated fats are more stable and far less prone to oxidation.) And of course, stay clear of the worst type of fat: trans fats, a.k.a. partially hydrogenated oils. These dangerous artificial fats are found in many processed foods, including commercial baked goods such as crackers, cookies, pies, and cakes; microwave popcorn; frozen pizza; stick margarine; fried foods such as French fries, doughnuts, and fried chicken; refrigerated doughs such as biscuits and rolls; and nondairy coffee creamers.

5) **Do not eat often**

   If you do nothing else, fast! Your body (including your muscles, of course) and your brain need clean-up and repair time. But there's no need to go without food for extended periods—you don't even need to fast for a full day. Time-restricted feeding (TRF) is the easiest and most popular form of intermittent fasting (IF). Eat within a window of 6 – 8 hours to allow for a fasting period of 16 – 18 hours. Do TRF daily or just a few days per week. Skipping breakfast is the easiest strategy for TRF, though you may prefer to skip dinner. (If you miss having breakfast foods, just eat them at lunch or dinner.) Simply delaying breakfast and/or eating an early dinner can work as well. However, it may be beneficial to cease eating around 3 hours before bedtime since late-night eating has been linked to poor health.

Upon beginning intermittent fasting, some people experience some mild to moderate adverse effects such as nausea, headache, insomnia, fatigue, and lightheadedness. *If you find fasting too difficult, follow a low-carbohydrate diet (fewer than 25% of your calories) for a few weeks first.* This will enable you to better burn fat and possibly ketones, thus helping you avoid carb/sugar cravings and dips in blood sugar.

6) **No need to count calories**

Constantly counting calories is totally unnecessary and rather burdensome. Calories count, of course, but they have different metabolic effects in the body depending on their source. Unless you're an aficionado of calorie-counting apps, for the sake of simplicity, just follow the guidelines outlined in this chapter.

7) **The most important supplements**

Among all of the muscle-enhancing supplements discussed in Chapter 10, *whey protein and creatine are at the top of the list*. Whey protein is the ideal post-workout food based on its superior anabolic properties, i.e., rapid digestion and rich leucine content. Take 20 – 30 grams of whey protein powder after exercising to optimize your muscle recovery and muscle protein synthesis. Older adults should consume a larger amount of about 40 grams due to anabolic resistance. If you use whey protein as a meal substitute, shoot for 30 – 50 grams.

Creatine is one of the most effective supplements for increasing muscle mass, strength, and power in both younger and older adults, particularly when combined with resistance training. A dosing strategy of 3 grams per day of creatine monohydrate (the most popular form) for 28 days will result in saturation of creatine in muscle and can be maintained over the long term. Another effective approach is loading about 5 grams of creatine monohydrate four times per day for 5 – 7 days, followed by a maintenance dosage of 3 – 5 grams/day.

I am putting three other supplements near the top as well: ***vitamin D, omega-3 fatty acids (EPA/DHA), and MCT oil.*** The reason I am giving high priority to vitamin D and fish oil supplements is that both go beyond muscle health—their shortage in the body is linked to a myriad of chronic degenerative diseases. Depending on your consumption of fatty fish such as tuna and salmon, take 2 – 4 grams per day of fish oil. These important omega-3 fats will activate your mTOR and sensitize your muscles to anabolic triggers (e.g., exercise, protein, insulin). They are even more important when you cannot be active.

In people with low levels of vitamin D, supplementation activates muscle protein synthesis. Vitamin D is also implicated in muscle damage repair and regeneration. I suggest higher-than-generally-recommended dosages of vitamin D3 (4,000 – 5,000 IU/day) combined with a mixture of 50 – 1,000 mcg/day of vitamins K1 and K2 (the latter prevent arterial calcification and vitamin D toxicity). These higher dosages of vitamin D correlate with the ideal blood levels that would be achieved if you had generous daily exposure to sunlight. Target having blood levels of 25-hydroxyvitamin D3 in the range of 50 – 70 ng/ml.

Supplementing with MCT oil is a simple and effective way to generate ketones without restricting carbs. Ketones spare muscle from being broken down for energy use. With higher ketone levels in your blood, you may experience sharper mental focus, better appetite control, increased fat loss, and, of course, better body composition. Ideally, add MCT oil to your post-workout whey protein beverage for an added boost to build/repair muscle tissue. Start with 1 teaspoon and build up to 3 teaspoons (which equals 1 tablespoon). You can also add MCT oil to foods such as scrambled eggs, yogurt, and salads. Choose a product with C8 MCT oil, as this variety churns out the most ketones.

An important caveat to close this section on supplements: *Avoid taking antioxidant supplements such as vitamin C, vitamin E, and beta-carotene around your workout!* Do not take them before exercising or within several hours after your workout. Why? Because paradoxically, exercise-induced free radicals are beneficial. Acute and transient exposure to these free radicals mediates some exercise adaptations, and these effects should not be suppressed by antioxidants.

8) **Take advantage of synergy**

Implementing at least some of each of the suggested interventions in this chapter provides synergistic benefits. A few examples:

1) High-quality dietary protein and resistance training act together to promote muscle protein synthesis better than either intervention alone, and they are both needed to actually *build muscle mass.*

2) Exercising on empty (fasting) will double down on depletion of muscle glycogen, which is linked to muscle protein synthesis and muscle growth. As a nice bonus, fat burning will be jacked up!

3) Fasting or taking MCT oil while on a very-low-carb diet will further boost ketone levels.

4) While resistance training alone improves cardiovascular fitness, adding HIIT to an RT regimen will only amplify cardio benefits.

To sum up and conclude, high-intensity interval training, fasting, low-carb eating, and certain nutritional supplements can contribute considerably to improving your muscle health and overall health. I highly recommend all of these powerful lifestyle interventions. Nevertheless, they are optional. You can certainly maintain your muscle mass and protect against muscle loss without them. On the other hand, when it comes to muscle health *exclusively*, **resistance exercise and high-quality animal protein** are non-negotiable. Don't go without them!

All roads lead to muscle! Disease and physical disability begin with the loss of muscle mass and strength and the deterioration of muscle quality. In a nutshell, while diminished ability to move around and function is a fairly obvious outcome of muscle loss, the link between chronic disease and muscle loss is not so obvious but easy to understand. Your body must maintain normal blood sugar levels because excess sugar in the blood is toxic to your cells. Muscle is essential to mop up and burn the excess sugar in your bloodstream. Loss of muscle and/or poor muscle quality resulting from lack of conditioning exercise - along with insufficient high-quality animal protein, excess carbs, and constant eating - impairs this process, leading to high blood sugar levels and potentially diabetes. Diabetes as well as prediabetes, in turn, significantly raise your risk of heart disease, cancer, Alzheimer's disease, osteoporosis, further muscle loss (sarcopenia), and accelerated aging.

Optimal muscle health means greater lifelong functionality, a lower risk of chronic diseases, and a longer healthspan. Functional aging is *not* inevitable. **Remember, we don't slow down because we're getting old—we get old because we slow down.**

Appendix

Sample Muscle Meals

Countless Paleo and keto cookbooks are filled with scrumptious recipes that adhere to the guidelines specified in Chapter 11. But for those of you who are not fond of spending a lot of time in the kitchen, here are some ideas for quick and easy meals that will go a long way toward supporting your muscle mass. Portions are given only for protein...hint, hint! (Protein is what really matters...)

Try to eat your starchy foods last, when you're almost full—that way, you'll eat less of them. In fact, eating most of your protein + veggies first and starches last significantly lowers the after-meal rise in blood sugar and insulin. And remember that breakfast can be eaten at any time of day to accommodate fasting. If you're on the keto plan, you may need to eliminate some of the fruit and starch portions so that your overall carb intake is about 50 grams or less.

As you browse through these suggestions, you'll see that I'm a huge avocado fan. Not only is avocado a superfood that's rich in potassium and healthful monounsaturated fats (particularly anti-aging oleic acid), eating avocadoes is a great way to get that "I'm full" feeling, thus lessening your need for carbs.

Breakfast Suggestions (eat any time of day)

- 4-egg omelet filled with 2 ounces of full-fat cheese, diced avocado, diced tomatoes, onions, and chopped garlic, all sautéed in extra-virgin olive oil (EVOO). You can add some mixed berries to this, too.
- ¾ cup full-fat plain Greek yogurt mixed with 1 scoop (about 25 grams) of chocolate whey protein powder, crushed walnuts, and berries.

- 6 – 8 ounces of ground turkey or turkey sausage sauteed with spinach, onions, avocado, and a generous splash of EVOO. Feel free to add slices of melon.
- High-protein breakfast smoothie: 1½ scoops of banana or chocolate whey protein powder (with about 37 grams of protein) plus ½ cup unsweetened almond milk, strawberries, and ½ cup full-fat plain Greek yogurt.
- 4 scrambled eggs with 4 strips of bacon, topped with pesto. You could add peach slices, too.
- 4 slices of smoked salmon with 2 ounces of aged Gouda cheese and some avocado. Try accompanying this with a tangerine.

Lunch & Dinner Suggestions

- 4 – 6 ounces grilled salmon, sweet potato, and broccoli with garlic and lemon.
- 8 – 12 ounces grilled pork loin porterhouse chop, green beans, corn on the cob with a mixed fruit salad.
- Large salad with tuna (4.5 ounces of canned tuna) and a variety of greens, tomatoes, mushrooms, onions, avocado, sprinkle of chopped walnuts, and ¼ cup full-fat shredded mozzarella cheese. Dress with a generous splash of EVOO along with apple cider vinegar to taste.
- 4-egg frittata with ¼ cup grated Romano cheese, zucchini, chopped onions, minced garlic, and parsley. Add ¾ cup full-fat plain Greek yogurt with berries on the side.
- 4 ounces roasted chicken breast with baked potato wedges and lemon-garlic roasted asparagus.
- 4 ounces full-fat Asiago or provolone cheese paired with fruit and a crushed walnut salad.

- 6 – 8 ounces beef tenderloin with grilled Brussels sprouts and red potatoes.
- 6 – 8 ounces of lamb chops with butternut squash and a spinach salad with apple slices, walnuts, and feta cheese.
- 4 – 6 ounces grilled trout with a Caesar salad. Add ¾ cup full-fat plain Greek yogurt with strawberries on the side.
- 4 – 6 ounces turkey tenderloin topped with avocado mayo, steamed vegetables, and mashed sweet potatoes.
- 100% whole-grain pasta with garlic and olive oil (*aglio e olio*) and 4 – 6 ounces beef sirloin tips.
- 4 – 6 ounces broiled calf liver topped with marinara sauce, mashed sweet potatoes, and zucchini sauteed in EVOO. Add ¾ cup full-fat plain Greek yogurt with berries on the side.

Common Non-Starchy Vegetables

- Artichoke
- Asparagus
- Beans (green, wax, Italian)
- Bean sprouts
- Beets
- Broccoli
- Cabbage (green, bok choy, Chinese)
- Carrots
- Cauliflower
- Celery
- Cucumber
- Daikon radish
- Eggplant
- Fennel
- Greens (lettuce, spinach, arugula, collard, kale, etc.)
- Hearts of palm
- Jicama
- Kohlrabi
- Leeks
- Mushrooms
- Okra
- Onions
- Pea pods
- Peppers

- Radishes
- Rutabaga
- Summer squash (yellow, zucchini)
- Tomatoes
- Turnips
- Water chestnuts

Common Low-Sugar Fruits

- Avocado
- Berries (all types)
- Cantaloupe
- Citrus (orange, grapefruit, lemon, lime)
- Honeydew melon
- Kiwi
- Peaches
- Plums
- Tart apples (e.g., Granny Smith)

Recommended Reading

1) *Sacred Cow* by Diana Rodgers and Robb Wolf.
   This an excellent read that debunks the myths about meat from nutritional, environmental, and ethical perspectives. If you want to understand why meat is good for you *and* the planet, then this is the book for you!

2) *The Carnivore Code* by Paul Saladino, MD.
   Like *Sacred Cow*, this outstanding book dives extensively into the controversy surrounding meat and—backed by science—shoots down all of the false claims that are misleading the general public today. When it comes eating meat, Dr. Saladino leaves no stone unturned.

3) *Body by Science* by Doug McGuff, MD, and John Little.
   This is my favorite book on fitness and exercise! The authors provide a unique perspective on the critical importance of high-intensity strength training, namely how it enhances your cardiovascular fitness. Though a bit technical, this book will explain the role of exercise in human health like no other. An eye-opening book and a must-read for all exercise enthusiasts.

4) *The Complete Guide to Fasting* by Jason Fung, MD, and Jimmy Moore.
   My favorite book on intermittent fasting! Dr. Jason Fung is one of the world's leading experts on this fascinating topic.

5) *The Art and Science of Low-Carbohydrate Living* by Jeff S. Volek and Stephen D. Phinney.
   Dr. Volek and Dr. Phinney are leading authorities on low-carbohydrate dieting.

6) *The Art and Science of Low-Carbohydrate Performance* by Jeff S. Volek and Stephen D. Phinney.
   The keto diet can benefit athletes as well. Another fascinating read.

7) *Eat Rich, Live Long* by Ivor Cummins and Jeffrey Gerber, MD.
   Another great book on why low-carb/keto diets are the best way to eat for optimal health and disease prevention. Very good discussion of insulin resistance. Bonus: fabulous low-carb recipes.

8) *The Ketogenic Bible* by Jacob Wilson and Ryan Lowery.
   Maybe the most comprehensive guide to ketosis. Awesome keto recipes.

9) *The Keto Reset Diet: Reboot Your Metabolism in 21 days and Burn Fat Forever* by Mark Sisson.
   Terrific best-selling book by a leading authority on the ketogenic diet. Delicious keto recipes included.

10) *The Obesity Code: Unlocking the Secrets of Weight Loss* by Jason Fung, MD.
   Another great book by Dr. Fung about how intermittent fasting and a low-carb/high-fat diet can promote permanent weight loss. Good explanation of how insulin and insulin resistance affect weight loss.

5 Basic Compound Exercises

For novice and non-bodybuilders, here are 5 basic compound exercises that should comprise the core of your fitness program. By targeting multiple muscle groups at one time, these compound exercises give you a time-efficient, full-body workout that will build muscle, increase strength, and improve cardiorespiratory fitness.

Squat (or Seated Leg Press)
Muscles worked: Gluteals, quadriceps, and hamstrings.

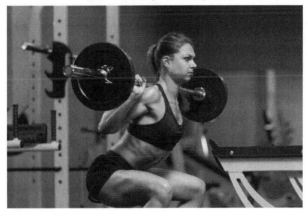

Copyright: satyrenko

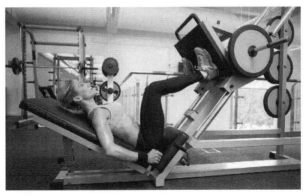

wavebreakmedia/shutterstock.com

Bench Press (or Chest Press Machine)

Muscles worked: Chest, shoulders, and triceps.

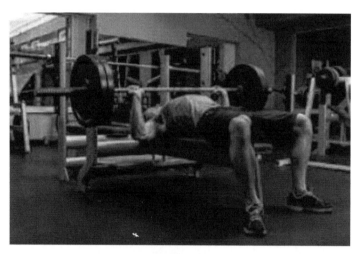

Copyright: ayphoto

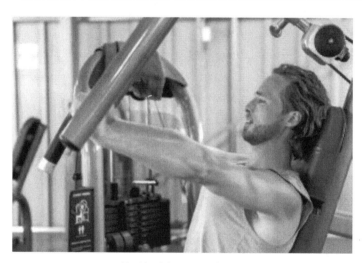

Maridav/shutterstock.com

Overhead Barbell/Dumbbell Press (or Overhead Press Machine)

Muscles worked: Anterior deltoids, triceps, and trapezius.

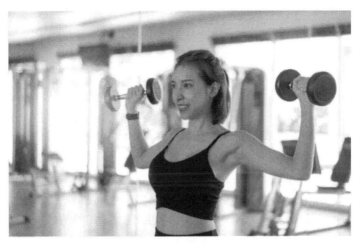

Copyright: marchsirawit

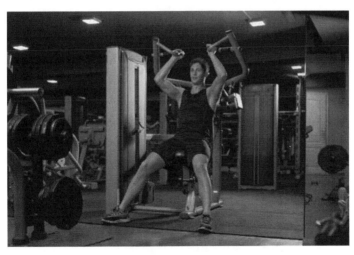

HD92/shutterstock.com

Barbell Row (or Seated Row/Lat Pulldown)

Muscles worked: Latissimus dorsi, rear deltoids, biceps, and upper back muscles around spine at base of neck.

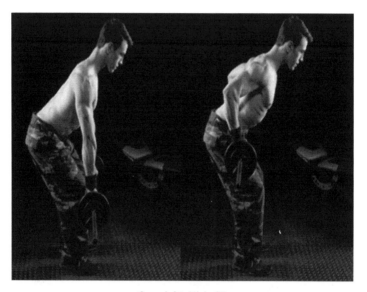

Copyright: Nickp37

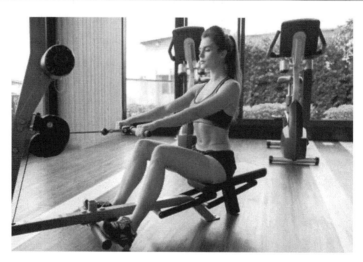

BLACKDAY/shutterstock.com

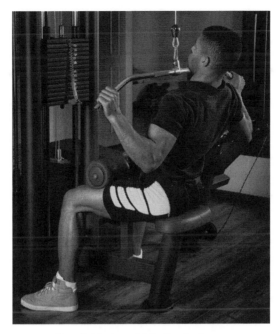

Copyright: starush/shutterstock.com

Dead Lift

Muscles worked: primarily quadriceps, gluteals, trapezius, and lower back.

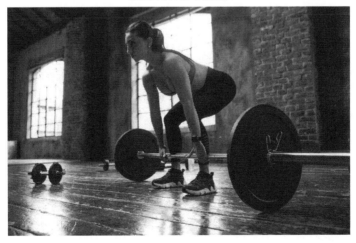

Copyright: oneinchpunch

References

Chapter 1

1. Srikanthan, P. and A.S. Karlamangla, *Muscle mass index as a predictor of longevity in older adults.* Am J Med, 2014. **127**(6): p. 547-53.

2. *CompX Research Institute. The Hypothesis.* 2016 2016 [cited 2020 08/05/2020]; Available from: https://www.compxtheory.com/the-hypothesis.

3. Tieland, M., I. Trouwborst, and B.C. Clark, *Skeletal muscle performance and ageing.* J Cachexia Sarcopenia Muscle, 2018. **9**(1): p. 3-19.

4. *Muscle: A Specialized Contractile Machine.*, in *Mlecular Cell Biology. 4th edition.*, B.A. Lodish H, Zipusky SL, et al. , Editor. 2000, W. H. Freeman: New York.

5. Dhillon, R.J. and S. Hasni, *Pathogenesis and Management of Sarcopenia.* Clin Geriatr Med, 2017. **33**(1): p. 17-26.

6. Chiles Shaffer, N., et al., *Muscle Quality, Strength, and Lower Extremity Physical Performance in the Baltimore Longitudinal Study of Aging.* J Frailty Aging, 2017. **6**(4): p. 183-187.

7. Robinson, S., A. Granic, and A.A. Sayer, *Nutrition and Muscle Strength, As the Key Component of Sarcopenia: An Overview of Current Evidence.* Nutrients, 2019. **11**(12).

8. Hunter, G.R., et al., *Sarcopenia and Its Implications for Metabolic Health.* J Obes, 2019. **2019**: p. 8031705.

9. Baskin, K.K., B.R. Winders, and E.N. Olson, *Muscle as a "mediator" of systemic metabolism.* Cell Metab, 2015. **21**(2): p. 237-248.

10. Mitchell, W.K., et al., *Sarcopenia, dynapenia, and the impact of advancing age on human skeletal muscle size and strength; a quantitative review.* Front Physiol, 2012. **3**: p. 260.

11. Hong, A.R. and S.W. Kim, *Effects of Resistance Exercise on Bone Health*. Endocrinol Metab (Seoul), 2018. **33**(4): p. 435-444.

12. Hirschfeld, H.P., R. Kinsella, and G. Duque, *Osteosarcopenia: where bone, muscle, and fat collide*. Osteoporos Int, 2017. **28**(10): p. 2781-2790.

13. Beaudart, C., et al., *Sarcopenia: burden and challenges for public health*. Arch Public Health, 2014. **72**(1): p. 45.

14. Pickering, M.E. and R. Chapurlat, *Where Two Common Conditions of Aging Meet: Osteoarthritis and Sarcopenia*. Calcif Tissue Int, 2020. **107**(3): p. 203-211.

15. Argilés, J.M., et al., *Skeletal Muscle Regulates Metabolism via Interorgan Crosstalk: Roles in Health and Disease*. Journal of the American Medical Directors Association, 2016. **17**(9): p. 789-796.

16. Wischmeyer, P.E., et al., *Muscle mass and physical recovery in ICU: innovations for targeting of nutrition and exercise*. Curr Opin Crit Care, 2017. **23**(4): p. 269-278.

17. Wischmeyer, P.E. and I. San-Millan, *Winning the war against ICU-acquired weakness: new innovations in nutrition and exercise physiology*. Crit Care, 2015. **19 Suppl 3**(Suppl 3): p. S6.

18. Beaudart C, Rolland Y, Cruz-Jentoft AJ, Bauer JM, Sieber C, Cooper C, Al-Daghri N, Araujo de Carvalho I, Bautmans I, Bernabei Ret al. Assessment of muscle function and physical performance in daily clinical practice: a position paper endorsed by the European Society for Clinical and Economic Aspects of Osteoporosis, Osteoarthritis and Musculoskeletal Diseases (ESCEO). *Calcif Tissue In*. 2019;105(1):1–14.

Chapter 2

1. Bhatti, J.S., G.K. Bhatti, and P.H. Reddy, *Mitochondrial dysfunction and oxidative stress in metabolic disorders - A step towards mitochondria based therapeutic strategies*. Biochimica et biophysica acta. Molecular basis of disease, 2017. **1863**(5): p. 1066-1077.

2. Sun, Y., et al., *Metabolism: A Novel Shared Link between Diabetes Mellitus and Alzheimer's Disease*. Journal of Diabetes Research, 2020. **2020**: p. 4981814.

3. Hotamisligil, G.S., *Inflammation and metabolic disorders*. Nature, 2006. **444**(7121): p. 860-7.

4. Araújo, J., J. Cai, and J. Stevens, *Prevalence of Optimal Metabolic Health in American Adults: National Health and Nutrition Examination Survey 2009-2016*. Metab Syndr Relat Disord, 2019. **17**(1): p. 46-52.

5. Graf, C. and N. Ferrari, *Metabolic Health-The Role of Adipo-Myokines*. Int J Mol Sci, 2019. **20**(24).

6. Kaminsky, L.A., et al., *The importance of cardiorespiratory fitness in the United States: the need for a national registry: a policy statement from the American Heart Association*. Circulation, 2013. **127**(5): p. 652-62.

7. Després, J.P., *Physical Activity, Sedentary Behaviours, and Cardiovascular Health: When Will Cardiorespiratory Fitness Become a Vital Sign?* Can J Cardiol, 2016. **32**(4): p. 505-13.

8. Biswas, A., et al., *Sedentary time and its association with risk for disease incidence, mortality, and hospitalization in adults: a systematic review and meta-analysis*. Ann Intern Med, 2015. **162**(2): p. 123-32.

9. Matthews, C.E., et al., *Mortality Benefits for Replacing Sitting Time with Different Physical Activities*. Med Sci Sports Exerc, 2015. **47**(9): p. 1833-40.

10. Ross, R., et al., *Importance of Assessing Cardiorespiratory Fitness in Clinical Practice: A Case for Fitness as a Clinical Vital Sign: A Scientific Statement From the American Heart Association*. Circulation, 2016. **134**(24): p. e653-e699.

11. Medicine, A.C.o.S., *ACSM's Guidelines for Exercise Testing and Prescription*. ninth ed. 2014: Wolters Kluwer Health/Lippincott Williams & Wilkins.

12. Stump, C.S., et al., *The metabolic syndrome: role of skeletal muscle metabolism*. Ann Med, 2006. **38**(6): p. 389-402.

13. Gim, M.N. and J.H. Choi, *The effects of weekly exercise time on VO2max and resting metabolic rate in normal adults*. J Phys Ther Sci, 2016. **28**(4): p. 1359-63.

14. Periasamy, M., J.L. Herrera, and F.C.G. Reis, *Skeletal Muscle Thermogenesis and Its Role in Whole Body Energy Metabolism.* Diabetes Metab J, 2017. **41**(5): p. 327-336.

15. Menke, A., et al., *Prevalence of and Trends in Diabetes Among Adults in the United States, 1988-2012.* JAMA, 2015. **314**(10): p. 1021-1029.

16. Saeedi, P., et al., *Global and regional diabetes prevalence estimates for 2019 and projections for 2030 and 2045: Results from the International Diabetes Federation Diabetes Atlas, 9(th) edition.* Diabetes Res Clin Pract, 2019. **157**: p. 107843.

17. Rowley, W.R., et al., *Diabetes 2030: Insights from Yesterday, Today, and Future Trends.* Popul Health Manag, 2017. **20**(1): p. 6-12.

18. Bertoluci, M.C. and V.Z. Rocha, *Cardiovascular risk assessment in patients with diabetes.* Diabetol Metab Syndr, 2017. **9**: p. 25.

19. Brutsaert, E.F. *Merck Manual Professional Version. Complications of Diabetes Mellitus.* September 2020 September 2020 [cited 2020 10/7/2020]; Available from: https://www.merckmanuals.com/professional/endocrine-and-metabolic-disorders/diabetes-mellitus-and-disorders-of-carbohydrate-metabolism/complications-of-diabetes-mellitus.

20. Petrie, J.R., T.J. Guzik, and R.M. Touyz, *Diabetes, Hypertension, and Cardiovascular Disease: Clinical Insights and Vascular Mechanisms.* Can J Cardiol, 2018. **34**(5): p. 575-584.

21. Fournet, M., F. Bonté, and A. Desmoulière, *Glycation Damage: A Possible Hub for Major Pathophysiological Disorders and Aging.* Aging Dis, 2018. **9**(5): p. 880-900.

22. *International Diabetes Federation. Abouit Diabetes. Diabetes facts & figures.* 2020 12/02/2020 [cited 2020 10/8/2020]; Available from: https://www.idf.org/aboutdiabetes/what-is-diabetes/facts-figures.html#:~:text=1%20in%202%20(232%20million,living%20with%20type%201%20diabetes.

23. Kalyani, R.R. and J.M. Egan, *Diabetes and altered glucose metabolism with aging.* Endocrinol Metab Clin North Am, 2013. **42**(2): p. 333-47.

24. Laiteerapong, N., et al., *The Legacy Effect in Type 2 Diabetes: Impact of Early Glycemic Control on Future Complications (The Diabetes & Aging Study)*. Diabetes Care, 2019. **42**(3): p. 416-426.

25. Sergi, D., et al., *The Role of Dietary Advanced Glycation End Products in Metabolic Dysfunction*. Mol Nutr Food Res, 2020: p. e1900934.

26. McCarty, M.F., *The low-AGE content of low-fat vegan diets could benefit diabetics - though concurrent taurine supplementation may be needed to minimize endogenous AGE production*. Med Hypotheses, 2005. **64**(2): p. 394-8.

27. Nowotny, K., et al., *Dietary advanced glycation end products and their relevance for human health*. Ageing Research Reviews, 2018. **47**: p. 55-66.

28. Ferrucci, L. and E. Fabbri, *Inflammageing: chronic inflammation in ageing, cardiovascular disease, and frailty*. Nat Rev Cardiol, 2018. **15**(9): p. 505-522.

29. Agrawal, N.K. and S. Kant, *Targeting inflammation in diabetes: Newer therapeutic options*. World J Diabetes, 2014. **5**(5): p. 697-710.

30. Singh, T. and A.B. Newman, *Inflammatory markers in population studies of aging*. Ageing Res Rev, 2011. **10**(3): p. 319-29.

31. Pomatto, L.C.D. and K.J.A. Davies, *Adaptive homeostasis and the free radical theory of ageing*. Free Radic Biol Med, 2018. **124**: p. 420-430.

32. Oguntibeju, O.O., *Type 2 diabetes mellitus, oxidative stress and inflammation: examining the links*. Int J Physiol Pathophysiol Pharmacol, 2019. **11**(3): p. 45-63.

33. Tan, B.L., et al., *Antioxidant and Oxidative Stress: A Mutual Interplay in Age-Related Diseases*. Front Pharmacol, 2018. **9**: p. 1162.

34. Biswas, S.K., *Does the Interdependence between Oxidative Stress and Inflammation Explain the Antioxidant Paradox?* Oxidative Medicine and Cellular Longevity, 2016. **2016**: p. 5698931.

35. Chadt, A. and H. Al-Hasani, *Glucose transporters in adipose tissue, liver, and skeletal muscle in metabolic health and disease*. Pflügers Archiv - European Journal of Physiology, 2020. **472**(9): p. 1273-1298.

36. Srikanthan, P. and A.S. Karlamangla, *Relative Muscle Mass Is Inversely Associated with Insulin Resistance and Prediabetes. Findings from The Third National Health and Nutrition Examination Survey.* The Journal of Clinical Endocrinology & Metabolism, 2011. **96**(9): p. 2898-2903.

37. Kirwan, J.P., J. Sacks, and S. Nieuwoudt, *The essential role of exercise in the management of type 2 diabetes.* Cleve Clin J Med, 2017. **84**(7 Suppl 1): p. S15-s21.

38. Anton, S.D., et al., *Flipping the Metabolic Switch: Understanding and Applying the Health Benefits of Fasting.* Obesity (Silver Spring), 2018. **26**(2): p. 254-268.

39. Kelley, D.E., *Skeletal muscle fat oxidation: timing and flexibility are everything.* J Clin Invest, 2005. **115**(7): p. 1699-702.

40. Kelley, D.E. and L.J. Mandarino, *Fuel selection in human skeletal muscle in insulin resistance: a reexamination.* Diabetes, 2000. **49**(5): p. 677-83.

41. Ormazabal, V., et al., *Association between insulin resistance and the development of cardiovascular disease.* Cardiovasc Diabetol, 2018. **17**(1): p. 122.

42. Astrup, A., et al., *Saturated Fats and Health: A Reassessment and Proposal for Food-Based Recommendations.* Journal of the American College of Cardiology, 2020. **76**(7): p. 844-857.

43. Smith, R.L., et al., *Metabolic Flexibility as an Adaptation to Energy Resources and Requirements in Health and Disease.* Endocr Rev, 2018. **39**(4): p. 489-517.

44. Diseases, N.N.I.o.D.a.D.a.K. *Overweight & Obesity Statistics.* 2017 August 2017 [cited 2021 8/23/2021]; Available from: https://www.niddk.nih.gov/health-information/health-statistics/overweight-obesity.

45. Bonora, E., et al., *Prevalence of insulin resistance in metabolic disorders: the Bruneck Study.* Diabetes, 1998. **47**(10): p. 1643-9.

46. Astrup, A., et al., *Saturated Fats and Health: A Reassessment and Proposal for Food-Based Recommendations: JACC State-of-the-Art Review.* J Am Coll Cardiol, 2020. **76**(7): p. 844-857.

47. Phinney, J.S.V.a.S.D., *The Art and Science of Low Carbohydrate Living.* 2011: Beyond Obesity LLC. 316.

48. Ukropcova, B., et al., *Dynamic changes in fat oxidation in human primary myocytes mirror metabolic characteristics of the donor.* J Clin Invest, 2005. **115**(7): p. 1934-41.

49. Phielix, E., et al., *High oxidative capacity due to chronic exercise training attenuates lipid-induced insulin resistance.* Diabetes, 2012. **61**(10): p. 2472-8.

50. Berggren, J.R., et al., *Skeletal muscle lipid oxidation and obesity: influence of weight loss and exercise.* Am J Physiol Endocrinol Metab, 2008. **294**(4): p. E726-32.

51. Rynders, C.A., et al., *Sedentary behaviour is a key determinant of metabolic inflexibility.* J Physiol, 2018. **596**(8): p. 1319-1330.

52. Severinsen, M.C.K. and B.K. Pedersen, *Muscle-Organ Crosstalk: The Emerging Roles of Myokines.* Endocr Rev, 2020. **41**(4): p. 594-609.

53. Son, J.S., et al., *Exercise-induced myokines: a brief review of controversial issues of this decade.* Expert Review of Endocrinology & Metabolism, 2018. **13**(1): p. 51-58.

54. Leal, L.G., M.A. Lopes, and M.L. Batista, Jr., *Physical Exercise-Induced Myokines and Muscle-Adipose Tissue Crosstalk: A Review of Current Knowledge and the Implications for Health and Metabolic Diseases.* Front Physiol, 2018. **9**: p. 1307.

55. Fischer, C.P., *Interleukin-6 in acute exercise and training: what is the biological relevance?* Exerc Immunol Rev, 2006. **12**: p. 6-33.

56. Schnyder, S. and C. Handschin, *Skeletal muscle as an endocrine organ: PGC-1α, myokines and exercise.* Bone, 2015. **80**: p. 115-125.

57. Rogeri, P.S., et al., *Crosstalk Between Skeletal Muscle and Immune System: Which Roles Do IL-6 and Glutamine Play?* Front Physiol, 2020. **11**: p. 582258.

58. Barbalho, S.M., et al., *Physical Exercise and Myokines: Relationships with Sarcopenia and Cardiovascular Complications.* Int J Mol Sci, 2020. **21**(10).

59. Hoffmann, C. and C. Weigert, *Skeletal Muscle as an Endocrine Organ: The Role of Myokines in Exercise Adaptations.* Cold Spring Harb Perspect Med, 2017. 7(11).

60. Tieland, M., I. Trouwborst, and B.C. Clark, *Skeletal muscle performance and ageing.* J Cachexia Sarcopenia Muscle, 2018. 9(1): p. 3-19.

61. Sleiman, S.F., et al., *Exercise promotes the expression of brain derived neurotrophic factor (BDNF) through the action of the ketone body β-hydroxybutyrate.* Elife, 2016. 5.

62. Yang, X., et al., *Muscle-generated BDNF is a sexually dimorphic myokine that controls metabolic flexibility.* Sci Signal, 2019. 12(594).

Chapter 3

1. Kokkinos, P. and J. Myers, *Exercise and physical activity: clinical outcomes and applications.* Circulation, 2010. 122(16): p. 1637-48.

2. Kalyani, R.R., M. Corriere, and L. Ferrucci, *Age-related and disease-related muscle loss: the effect of diabetes, obesity, and other diseases.* Lancet Diabetes Endocrinol, 2014. 2(10): p. 819-29.

3. Booth, F.W., C.K. Roberts, and M.J. Laye, *Lack of exercise is a major cause of chronic diseases.* Compr Physiol, 2012. 2(2): p. 1143-211.

4. Breen, L., et al., *Two weeks of reduced activity decreases leg lean mass and induces "anabolic resistance" of myofibrillar protein synthesis in healthy elderly.* J Clin Endocrinol Metab, 2013. 98(6): p. 2604-12.

5. Booth, F.W., M.V. Chakravarthy, and E.E. Spangenburg, *Exercise and gene expression: physiological regulation of the human genome through physical activity.* J Physiol, 2002. 543(Pt 2): p. 399-411.

6. Bouchard, C., S.N. Blair, and P.T. Katzmarzyk, *Less Sitting, More Physical Activity, or Higher Fitness?* Mayo Clin Proc, 2015. 90(11): p. 1533-40.

7. Frontera, W.R. and J. Ochala, *Skeletal muscle: a brief review of structure and function.* Calcif Tissue Int, 2015. 96(3): p. 183-95.

8. Bell, K.E., et al., *Muscle Disuse as a Pivotal Problem in Sarcopenia-related Muscle Loss and Dysfunction.* J Frailty Aging, 2016. **5**(1): p. 33-41.

9. Timmerman, K.L., et al., *Pharmacological vasodilation improves insulin-stimulated muscle protein anabolism but not glucose utilization in older adults.* Diabetes, 2010. **59**(11): p. 2764-71.

10. Lawler, J.M. and A. Hindle, *Living in a box or call of the wild? Revisiting lifetime inactivity and sarcopenia.* Antioxid Redox Signal, 2011. **15**(9): p. 2529-41.

Chapter 4

1. Kuipers, R.S., et al., *Estimated macronutrient and fatty acid intakes from an East African Paleolithic diet.* Br J Nutr, 2010. **104**(11): p. 1666-87.

2. Agriculture, U.D.o.H.a.H.S.a.U.D.o., *2015-2020 Dietary Guidelines for Americans*, U.a. HHS, Editor. 2015.

3. Jung, C.H. and K.M. Choi, *Impact of High-Carbohydrate Diet on Metabolic Parameters in Patients with Type 2 Diabetes.* Nutrients, 2017. **9**(4).

4. Oh, R., B. Gilani, and K.R. Uppaluri, *Low Carbohydrate Diet*, in *StatPearls*. 2020, StatPearls Publishing Copyright © 2020, StatPearls Publishing LLC.: Treasure Island (FL).

5. Ludwig, D.S., et al., *Dietary carbohydrates: role of quality and quantity in chronic disease.* Bmj, 2018. **361**: p. k2340.

6. Paoli, A., et al., *Ketogenic Diet and Skeletal Muscle Hypertrophy: A Frenemy Relationship?* J Hum Kinet, 2019. **68**: p. 233-247.

7. Ströhle, A. and A. Hahn, *Diets of modern hunter-gatherers vary substantially in their carbohydrate content depending on ecoenvironments: results from an ethnographic analysis.* Nutr Res, 2011. **31**(6): p. 429-35.

8. O'Keefe, J.H., Jr. and L. Cordain, *Cardiovascular disease resulting from a diet and lifestyle at odds with our Paleolithic genome: how*

to become a 21st-century hunter-gatherer. Mayo Clin Proc, 2004. **79**(1): p. 101-8.

9. Saniotis, A., M. Henneberg, and D. Olney, *Curse of Carbohydrate: How the Rise of Agriculturalism Led to the Demise of Homo.* Human Evolution, 2020. **34**: p. 133-138.

10. DiNicolantonio, J.J. and J.H. O'Keefe, *The introduction of refined carbohydrates in the Alaskan Inland Inuit diet may have led to an increase in dental caries, hypertension and atherosclerosis.* Open Heart, 2018. **5**(2): p. e000776.

11. Kopp, W., *How Western Diet And Lifestyle Drive The Pandemic Of Obesity And Civilization Diseases.* Diabetes Metab Syndr Obes, 2019. **12**: p. 2221-2236.

12. Pontzer, H., B.M. Wood, and D.A. Raichlen, *Hunter-gatherers as models in public health.* Obesity Reviews, 2018. **19**(S1): p. 24-35.

13. Spreadbury, I., *Comparison with ancestral diets suggests dense acellular carbohydrates promote an inflammatory microbiota, and may be the primary dietary cause of leptin resistance and obesity.* Diabetes Metab Syndr Obes, 2012. **5**: p. 175-89.

14. Buettner, D. and S. Skemp, *Blue Zones: Lessons From the World's Longest Lived.* Am J Lifestyle Med, 2016. **10**(5): p. 318-321.

15. Dehghan, M., et al., *Associations of fats and carbohydrate intake with cardiovascular disease and mortality in 18 countries from five continents (PURE): a prospective cohort study.* Lancet, 2017. **390**(10107): p. 2050-2062.

16. Hariton, E. and J.J. Locascio, *Randomised controlled trials - the gold standard for effectiveness research: Study design: randomised controlled trials.* Bjog, 2018. **125**(13): p. 1716.

17. Bhanpuri, N.H., et al., *Cardiovascular disease risk factor responses to a type 2 diabetes care model including nutritional ketosis induced by sustained carbohydrate restriction at 1 year: an open label, non-randomized, controlled study.* Cardiovasc Diabetol, 2018. **17**(1): p. 56.

18. Santos, F.L., et al., *Systematic review and meta-analysis of clinical trials of the effects of low carbohydrate diets on cardiovascular risk factors.* Obes Rev, 2012. **13**(11): p. 1048-66.

19. Dong, T., et al., *The effects of low-carbohydrate diets on cardiovascular risk factors: A meta-analysis.* PLoS One, 2020. **15**(1): p. e0225348.

20. Mansoor, N., et al., *Effects of low-carbohydrate diets v. low-fat diets on body weight and cardiovascular risk factors: a meta-analysis of randomised controlled trials.* Br J Nutr, 2016. **115**(3): p. 466-79.

21. Bueno, N.B., et al., *Very-low-carbohydrate ketogenic diet v. low-fat diet for long-term weight loss: a meta-analysis of randomised controlled trials.* Br J Nutr, 2013. **110**(7): p. 1178-87.

22. Tobias, D.K., et al., *Effect of low-fat diet interventions versus other diet interventions on long-term weight change in adults: a systematic review and meta-analysis.* Lancet Diabetes Endocrinol, 2015. **3**(12): p. 968-79.

23. Davies, M.J., et al., *Management of Hyperglycemia in Type 2 Diabetes, 2018. A Consensus Report by the American Diabetes Association (ADA) and the European Association for the Study of Diabetes (EASD).* Diabetes Care, 2018. **41**(12): p. 2669-2701.

24. Lasker, D.A., E.M. Evans, and D.K. Layman, *Moderate carbohydrate, moderate protein weight loss diet reduces cardiovascular disease risk compared to high carbohydrate, low protein diet in obese adults: A randomized clinical trial.* Nutr Metab (Lond), 2008. **5**: p. 30.

25. Layman, D.K., et al., *A reduced ratio of dietary carbohydrate to protein improves body composition and blood lipid profiles during weight loss in adult women.* J Nutr, 2003. **133**(2): p. 411-7.

26. Devkota, S. and D.K. Layman, *Increased ratio of dietary carbohydrate to protein shifts the focus of metabolic signaling from skeletal muscle to adipose.* Nutr Metab (Lond), 2011. **8**(1): p. 13.

27. Schiaffino, S. and C. Mammucari, *Regulation of skeletal muscle growth by the IGF1-Akt/PKB pathway: insights from genetic models.* Skeletal Muscle, 2011. **1**(1): p. 4.

28. Furuichi, Y., et al., *Excess Glucose Impedes the Proliferation of Skeletal Muscle Satellite Cells Under Adherent Culture Conditions.* Front Cell Dev Biol, 2021. **9**: p. 640399.

Chapter 5

1. Fujita, S., et al., *Nutrient signalling in the regulation of human muscle protein synthesis.* J Physiol, 2007. **582**(Pt 2): p. 813-23.
2. Layman, D.K., et al., *Defining meal requirements for protein to optimize metabolic roles of amino acids.* The American Journal of Clinical Nutrition, 2015. **101**(6): p. 1330S-1338S.
3. Layman, D.K., *Dietary Guidelines should reflect new understandings about adult protein needs.* Nutr Metab (Lond), 2009. **6**: p. 12.
4. Bauer, J., et al., *Evidence-based recommendations for optimal dietary protein intake in older people: a position paper from the PROT-AGE Study Group.* J Am Med Dir Assoc, 2013. **14**(8): p. 542-59.
5. Wu, G., *Dietary protein intake and human health.* Food Funct, 2016. **7**(3): p. 1251-65.
6. Yoon, M.S., *mTOR as a Key Regulator in Maintaining Skeletal Muscle Mass.* Front Physiol, 2017. **8**: p. 788.
7. Richter, M., et al., *Revised Reference Values for the Intake of Protein.* Ann Nutr Metab, 2019. **74**(3): p. 242-250.
8. Wolfe, R.R., et al., *Optimizing Protein Intake in Adults: Interpretation and Application of the Recommended Dietary Allowance Compared with the Acceptable Macronutrient Distribution Range.* Adv Nutr, 2017. **8**(2): p. 266-275.
9. Phillips, S.M., D. Paddon-Jones, and D.K. Layman, *Optimizing Adult Protein Intake During Catabolic Health Conditions.* Adv Nutr, 2020. **11**(4): p. S1058-s1069.
10. Mamerow, M.M., et al., *Dietary protein distribution positively influences 24-h muscle protein synthesis in healthy adults.* J Nutr, 2014. **144**(6): p. 876-80.
11. Atherton, P.J. and K. Smith, *Muscle protein synthesis in response to nutrition and exercise.* J Physiol, 2012. **590**(5): p. 1049-57.

12. Stokes, T., et al., *Recent Perspectives Regarding the Role of Dietary Protein for the Promotion of Muscle Hypertrophy with Resistance Exercise Training.* Nutrients, 2018. **10**(2).

13. Hevia-Larraín, V., et al., *High-Protein Plant-Based Diet Versus a Protein-Matched Omnivorous Diet to Support Resistance Training Adaptations: A Comparison Between Habitual Vegans and Omnivores.* Sports Med, 2021. **51**(6): p. 1317-1330.

14. Reidy, P.T. and B.B. Rasmussen, *Role of Ingested Amino Acids and Protein in the Promotion of Resistance Exercise-Induced Muscle Protein Anabolism.* J Nutr, 2016. **146**(2): p. 155-83.

15. Devries, M. and S. Phillips, *Supplemental Protein in Support of Muscle Mass and Health: Advantage Whey.* Journal of Food Science, 2015. **80**.

16. Aragon, A.A. and B.J. Schoenfeld, *Nutrient timing revisited: is there a post-exercise anabolic window?* J Int Soc Sports Nutr, 2013. **10**(1): p. 5.

17. Areta, J.L., et al., *Timing and distribution of protein ingestion during prolonged recovery from resistance exercise alters myofibrillar protein synthesis.* The Journal of Physiology, 2013. **591**(9): p. 2319-2331.

18. Davies, R.W., B.P. Carson, and P.M. Jakeman, *The Effect of Whey Protein Supplementation on the Temporal Recovery of Muscle Function Following Resistance Training: A Systematic Review and Meta-Analysis.* Nutrients, 2018. **10**(2).

19. Lam, F.C., et al., *Effectiveness of whey protein supplements on the serum levels of amino acid, creatinine kinase and myoglobin of athletes: a systematic review and meta-analysis.* Syst Rev, 2019. **8**(1): p. 130.

20. Yang, Y., et al., *Resistance exercise enhances myofibrillar protein synthesis with graded intakes of whey protein in older men.* Br J Nutr, 2012. **108**(10): p. 1780-8.

21. Ferrando, A.A., et al., *EAA supplementation to increase nitrogen intake improves muscle function during bed rest in the elderly.* Clin Nutr, 2010. **29**(1): p. 18-23.

22. Staples, A.W., et al., *Carbohydrate does not augment exercise-induced protein accretion versus protein alone.* Med Sci Sports Exerc, 2011. **43**(7): p. 1154-61.

23. Evans, M., K.E. Cogan, and B. Egan, *Metabolism of ketone bodies during exercise and training: physiological basis for exogenous supplementation.* J Physiol, 2017. **595**(9): p. 2857-2871.

24. Volek, J.S., et al., *Metabolic characteristics of keto-adapted ultra-endurance runners.* Metabolism, 2016. **65**(3): p. 100-10.

25. Robergs, R.A., et al., *Muscle glycogenolysis during differing intensities of weight-resistance exercise.* J Appl Physiol (1985), 1991. **70**(4): p. 1700-6.

26. Layman, D.K., *Assessing the Role of Cattle in Sustainable Food Systems.* Nutrition Today, 2018. **53**(4): p. 160-165.

27. Berrazaga, I., et al., *The Role of the Anabolic Properties of Plant- versus Animal-Based Protein Sources in Supporting Muscle Mass Maintenance: A Critical Review.* Nutrients, 2019. **11**(8).

28. Norton, L.E., et al., *The leucine content of a complete meal directs peak activation but not duration of skeletal muscle protein synthesis and mammalian target of rapamycin signaling in rats.* J Nutr, 2009. **139**(6): p. 1103-9.

29. Yang, Y., et al., *Myofibrillar protein synthesis following ingestion of soy protein isolate at rest and after resistance exercise in elderly men.* Nutrition & Metabolism, 2012. **9**(1): p. 57.

30. Hackney, K.J., et al., *Protein and muscle health during aging: benefits and concerns related to animal-based protein.* Anim Front, 2019. **9**(4): p. 12-17.

31. Wu, G., *Important roles of dietary taurine, creatine, carnosine, anserine and 4-hydroxyproline in human nutrition and health.* Amino Acids, 2020. **52**(3): p. 329-360.

32. Varanoske, A.N., et al., *Influence of Skeletal Muscle Carnosine Content on Fatigue during Repeated Resistance Exercise in Recreationally Active Women.* Nutrients, 2017. **9**(9).

33. White, R.R. and M.B. Hall, *Nutritional and greenhouse gas impacts of removing animals from US agriculture.* Proc Natl Acad Sci U S A, 2017. **114**(48): p. E10301-e10308.

34. Ben-Dor, M., R. Sirtoli, and R. Barkai, *The evolution of the human trophic level during the Pleistocene.* Am J Phys Anthropol, 2021. **175 Suppl 72**: p. 27-56.

35. McKendry, J., et al., *Nutritional Supplements to Support Resistance Exercise in Countering the Sarcopenia of Aging.* Nutrients, 2020. **12**(7).

36. Gibson, M.J., et al., *A randomized cross-over trial to determine the effect of a protein vs. carbohydrate preload on energy balance in ad libitum settings.* Nutr J, 2019. **18**(1): p. 69.

Chapter 6

1. Drummond, M.J., et al., *Skeletal muscle protein anabolic response to resistance exercise and essential amino acids is delayed with aging.* J Appl Physiol (1985), 2008. **104**(5): p. 1452-61.

2. Layman, D.K., et al., *Defining meal requirements for protein to optimize metabolic roles of amino acids.* The American Journal of Clinical Nutrition, 2015. **101**(6): p. 1330S-1338S.

3. Bauer, J., et al., *Evidence-based recommendations for optimal dietary protein intake in older people: a position paper from the PROT-AGE Study Group.* J Am Med Dir Assoc, 2013. **14**(8): p. 542-59.

4. Marshall, R.N., et al., *Nutritional Strategies to Offset Disuse-Induced Skeletal Muscle Atrophy and Anabolic Resistance in Older Adults: From Whole-Foods to Isolated Ingredients.* Nutrients, 2020. **12**(5).

5. Barclay, R.D., et al., *The Role of the IGF-1 Signaling Cascade in Muscle Protein Synthesis and Anabolic Resistance in Aging Skeletal Muscle.* Front Nutr, 2019. **6**: p. 146.

6. Wall, B.T., et al., *Short-term muscle disuse lowers myofibrillar protein synthesis rates and induces anabolic resistance to protein ingestion.* Am J Physiol Endocrinol Metab, 2016. **310**(2): p. E137-47.

7. Symons, T.B., et al., *Aging does not impair the anabolic response to a protein-rich meal.* Am J Clin Nutr, 2007. **86**(2): p. 451-6.

8. Moro, T., et al., *Muscle Protein Anabolic Resistance to Essential Amino Acids Does Not Occur in Healthy Older Adults Before or After Resistance Exercise Training.* J Nutr, 2018. **148**(6): p. 900-909.

9. Shad, B.J., J.L. Thompson, and L. Breen, *Does the muscle protein synthetic response to exercise and amino acid-based nutrition diminish with advancing age? A systematic review.* Am J Physiol Endocrinol Metab, 2016. **311**(5): p. E803-e817.

10. Moore, D.R., et al., *Differential stimulation of myofibrillar and sarcoplasmic protein synthesis with protein ingestion at rest and after resistance exercise.* J Physiol, 2009. **587**(Pt 4): p. 897-904.

11. Saxton, R.A. and D.M. Sabatini, *mTOR Signaling in Growth, Metabolism, and Disease.* Cell, 2017. **168**(6): p. 960-976.

12. Menzies, F.M., et al., *Autophagy and Neurodegeneration: Pathogenic Mechanisms and Therapeutic Opportunities.* Neuron, 2017. **93**(5): p. 1015-1034.

13. Park, S.S., Y.K. Seo, and K.S. Kwon, *Sarcopenia targeting with autophagy mechanism by exercise.* BMB Rep, 2019. **52**(1): p. 64-69.

14. Li, S., et al., *Excessive Autophagy Activation and Increased Apoptosis Are Associated with Palmitic Acid-Induced Cardiomyocyte Insulin Resistance.* J Diabetes Res, 2017. **2017**: p. 2376893.

15. Yerbury, J.J., et al., *Walking the tightrope: proteostasis and neurodegenerative disease.* J Neurochem, 2016. **137**(4): p. 489-505.

16. Beals, J.W., et al., *Anabolic sensitivity of postprandial muscle protein synthesis to the ingestion of a protein-dense food is reduced in overweight and obese young adults.* Am J Clin Nutr, 2016. **104**(4): p. 1014-1022.

17. Beals, J.W., et al., *Obesity Alters the Muscle Protein Synthetic Response to Nutrition and Exercise.* Frontiers in Nutrition, 2019. **6**(87).

18. Moore, D.R., et al., *Protein ingestion to stimulate myofibrillar protein synthesis requires greater relative protein intakes in healthy older versus younger men.* J Gerontol A Biol Sci Med Sci, 2015. **70**(1): p. 57-62.

19. Morton, R., et al., *Defining anabolic resistance: Implications for delivery of clinical care nutrition.* Current Opinion in Critical Care, 2018. **24**: p. 1.

20. Breen, L. and S.M. Phillips, *Skeletal muscle protein metabolism in the elderly: Interventions to counteract the 'anabolic resistance' of ageing.* Nutr Metab (Lond), 2011. **8**: p. 68.

Chapter 7

1. Booth, F.W., M.V. Chakravarthy, and E.E. Spangenburg, *Exercise and gene expression: physiological regulation of the human genome through physical activity.* J Physiol, 2002. **543**(Pt 2): p. 399-411.
2. Bell, K.E., et al., *Day-to-Day Changes in Muscle Protein Synthesis in Recovery From Resistance, Aerobic, and High-Intensity Interval Exercise in Older Men.* J Gerontol A Biol Sci Med Sci, 2015. **70**(8): p. 1024-9.
3. Sculthorpe, N.F., P. Herbert, and F. Grace, *One session of high-intensity interval training (HIIT) every 5 days, improves muscle power but not static balance in lifelong sedentary ageing men: A randomized controlled trial.* Medicine (Baltimore), 2017. **96**(6): p. e6040.
4. Robinson, M.M., et al., *Enhanced Protein Translation Underlies Improved Metabolic and Physical Adaptations to Different Exercise Training Modes in Young and Old Humans.* Cell Metab, 2017. **25**(3): p. 581-592.
5. McLeod, J.C., T. Stokes, and S.M. Phillips, *Resistance Exercise Training as a Primary Countermeasure to Age-Related Chronic Disease.* Front Physiol, 2019. **10**: p. 645.
6. Shaw, B., I. Shaw, and G. Brown, *Resistance exercise is medicine: Strength training in health promotion and rehabilitation.* International Journal of Therapy and Rehabilitation, 2015. **22**: p. 385-389.
7. Melov, S., et al., *Resistance exercise reverses aging in human skeletal muscle.* PLoS One, 2007. **2**(5): p. e465.
8. Lee, I.M. and R.S. Paffenbarger, Jr., *Associations of light, moderate, and vigorous intensity physical activity with longevity. The Harvard Alumni Health Study.* Am J Epidemiol, 2000. **151**(3): p. 293-9.

9. Kincaid, B. and E. Bossy-Wetzel, *Forever young: SIRT3 a shield against mitochondrial meltdown, aging, and neurodegeneration.* Frontiers in Aging Neuroscience, 2013. **5**.

10. Lee, S.H., et al., *Sirtuin signaling in cellular senescence and aging.* BMB Rep, 2019. **52**(1): p. 24-34.

11. Das, A., et al., *Impairment of an Endothelial NAD+-H2S Signaling Network Is a Reversible Cause of Vascular Aging.* Cell, 2018. **173**(1): p. 74-89.e20.

12. El Hayek, L., et al., *Lactate Mediates the Effects of Exercise on Learning and Memory through SIRT1-Dependent Activation of Hippocampal Brain-Derived Neurotrophic Factor (BDNF).* The Journal of Neuroscience, 2019. **39**(13): p. 2369-2382.

13. Damas, F., et al., *Resistance training-induced changes in integrated myofibrillar protein synthesis are related to hypertrophy only after attenuation of muscle damage.* J Physiol, 2016. **594**(18): p. 5209-22.

14. Lloyd, R.S., et al., *Position statement on youth resistance training: the 2014 International Consensus.* Br J Sports Med, 2014. **48**(7): p. 498-505.

15. Hawley, J.A., et al., *Integrative biology of exercise.* Cell, 2014. **159**(4): p. 738-49.

16. Morton, R., C. McGlory, and S. Phillips, *Nutritional interventions to augment resistance training-induced skeletal muscle hypertrophy.* Frontiers in Physiology, 2015. **6**(245).

17. Hart, P.D. and D.J. Buck, *The effect of resistance training on health-related quality of life in older adults: Systematic review and meta-analysis.* Health Promot Perspect, 2019. **9**(1): p. 1-12.

18. Westcott, W.L., *BUILD MUSCLE, IMPROVE HEALTH: BENEFITS ASSOCIATED WITH RESISTANCE EXERCISE.* ACSM's Health & Fitness Journal, 2015. **19**(4): p. 22-27.

19. *American College of Sports Medicine position stand. Progression models in resistance training for healthy adults.* Med Sci Sports Exerc, 2009. **41**(3): p. 687-708.

20. Garber, C.E., et al., *American College of Sports Medicine position stand. Quantity and quality of exercise for developing and*

maintaining cardiorespiratory, musculoskeletal, and neuromotor fitness in apparently healthy adults: guidance for prescribing exercise. Med Sci Sports Exerc, 2011. **43**(7): p. 1334-59.

21. Piercy, K.L., et al., *The Physical Activity Guidelines for Americans.* Jama, 2018. **320**(19): p. 2020-2028.

22. Morton, R.W., L. Colenso-Semple, and S.M. Phillips, *Training for strength and hypertrophy: an evidence-based approach.* Current Opinion in Physiology, 2019. **10**: p. 90-95.

23. Grgic, J., et al., *Effects of Rest Interval Duration in Resistance Training on Measures of Muscular Strength: A Systematic Review.* Sports Medicine, 2018. **48**(1): p. 137-151.

24. Burd, N.A., et al., *Bigger weights may not beget bigger muscles: evidence from acute muscle protein synthetic responses after resistance exercise.* Appl Physiol Nutr Metab, 2012. **37**(3): p. 551-4.

25. Phillips, S.M. and R.A. Winett, *Uncomplicated resistance training and health-related outcomes: evidence for a public health mandate.* Curr Sports Med Rep, 2010. **9**(4): p. 208-13.

26. Morton, R.W., et al., *Muscle fibre activation is unaffected by load and repetition duration when resistance exercise is performed to task failure.* J Physiol, 2019. **597**(17): p. 4601-4613.

27. McGuff, D. and J.R. Little, *Body by science : a research based program to get the results you want in 12 minutes a week.* 2009, New York: McGraw-Hill.

28. Sato, S., et al., *Effect of daily 3-s maximum voluntary isometric, concentric, or eccentric contraction on elbow flexor strength.* Scandinavian Journal of Medicine & Science in Sports. **n/a**(n/a).

29. Mukund, K. and S. Subramaniam, *Skeletal muscle: A review of molecular structure and function, in health and disease.* Wiley Interdiscip Rev Syst Biol Med, 2020. **12**(1): p. e1462.

30. Ogborn, D. and B.J. Schoenfeld, *The Role of Fiber Types in Muscle Hypertrophy: Implications for Loading Strategies.* Strength & Conditioning Journal, 2014. **36**(2): p. 20-25.

31. Siparsky, P.N., D.T. Kirkendall, and W.E. Garrett, Jr., *Muscle changes in aging: understanding sarcopenia.* Sports Health, 2014. **6**(1): p. 36-40.

32. Kramer, I.F., et al., *Extensive Type II Muscle Fiber Atrophy in Elderly Female Hip Fracture Patients.* J Gerontol A Biol Sci Med Sci, 2017. **72**(10): p. 1369-1375.

33. Frontera, W.R., et al., *Strength conditioning in older men: skeletal muscle hypertrophy and improved function.* J Appl Physiol (1985), 1988. **64**(3): p. 1038-44.

34. Fiatarone, M.A., et al., *High-intensity strength training in nonagenarians. Effects on skeletal muscle.* Jama, 1990. **263**(22): p. 3029-34.

35. Hearris, M.A., et al., *Regulation of Muscle Glycogen Metabolism during Exercise: Implications for Endurance Performance and Training Adaptations.* Nutrients, 2018. **10**(3).

36. Baker, J.S., M.C. McCormick, and R.A. Robergs, *Interaction among Skeletal Muscle Metabolic Energy Systems during Intense Exercise.* J Nutr Metab, 2010. **2010**: p. 905612.

37. Murray, B. and C. Rosenbloom, *Fundamentals of glycogen metabolism for coaches and athletes.* Nutr Rev, 2018. **76**(4): p. 243-259.

38. Jensen, J., et al., *The Role of Skeletal Muscle Glycogen Breakdown for Regulation of Insulin Sensitivity by Exercise.* Frontiers in physiology, 2011. **2**: p. 112.

39. Bartlett, J.D., J.A. Hawley, and J.P. Morton, *Carbohydrate availability and exercise training adaptation: too much of a good thing?* Eur J Sport Sci, 2015. **15**(1): p. 3-12.

40. Hulston, C.J., et al., *Training with low muscle glycogen enhances fat metabolism in well-trained cyclists.* Med Sci Sports Exerc, 2010. **42**(11): p. 2046-55.

41. Joseph, A.M., P.J. Adhihetty, and C. Leeuwenburgh, *Beneficial effects of exercise on age-related mitochondrial dysfunction and oxidative stress in skeletal muscle.* J Physiol, 2016. **594**(18): p. 5105-23.

42. Richter, E.A., W. Derave, and J.F. Wojtaszewski, *Glucose, exercise and insulin: emerging concepts.* J Physiol, 2001. **535**(Pt 2): p. 313-22.

43. Petersen, K.F., et al., *The role of skeletal muscle insulin resistance in the pathogenesis of the metabolic syndrome.* Proc Natl Acad Sci U S A, 2007. **104**(31): p. 12587-94.

44. Testoni, G., et al., *Lack of Glycogenin Causes Glycogen Accumulation and Muscle Function Impairment.* Cell Metabolism, 2017. **26**(1): p. 256-266.e4.

45. Rynders, C.A., et al., *Effects of Exercise Intensity on Postprandial Improvement in Glucose Disposal and Insulin Sensitivity in Prediabetic Adults.* The Journal of Clinical Endocrinology & Metabolism, 2014. **99**(1): p. 220-228.

46. Steele, J., J.J. Fisher, and S. Bruce-Low. *Resistance Training to Momentary Muscular Failure Improves Cardiovascular Fitness in Humans: A Review of Acute Physiological Responses and Chronic Physiological Adaptations.* 2012.

47. Smith, M.P., *Independent cardioprotective effects of resistance and aerobic exercise training in adults.* Eur J Prev Cardiol, 2020. **27**(19): p. 2226-2228.

48. Brooks, G.A., *Cell-cell and intracellular lactate shuttles.* J Physiol, 2009. **587**(Pt 23): p. 5591-600.

49. Nalbandian, M. and M. Takeda, *Lactate as a Signaling Molecule That Regulates Exercise-Induced Adaptations.* Biology (Basel), 2016. **5**(4).

50. Kyun, S., et al., *The Effects of Exogenous Lactate Administration on the IGF1/Akt/mTOR Pathway in Rat Skeletal Muscle.* Int J Environ Res Public Health, 2020. 17(21).

51. Murawska-Ciałowicz, E., et al., *Effect of four different forms of high intensity training on BDNF response to Wingate and Graded Exercise Test.* Sci Rep, 2021. **11**(1): p. 8599.

52. Ohno, Y., et al., *Lactate Stimulates a Potential for Hypertrophy and Regeneration of Mouse Skeletal Muscle.* Nutrients, 2019. **11**(4).

53. Schleppenbach, L.N., et al., *Speed- and Circuit-Based High-Intensity Interval Training on Recovery Oxygen Consumption.* Int J Exerc Sci, 2017. **10**(7): p. 942-953.

54. Panissa, V.L.G., et al., *Magnitude and duration of excess of post-exercise oxygen consumption between high-intensity interval and moderate-intensity continuous exercise: A systematic review.* Obes Rev, 2021. **22**(1): p. e13099.

55. Hackney, K.J., H.J. Engels, and R.J. Gretebeck, *Resting energy expenditure and delayed-onset muscle soreness after full-body resistance training with an eccentric concentration.* J Strength Cond Res, 2008. **22**(5): p. 1602-9.

56. Tang, J.E., J.W. Hartman, and S.M. Phillips, *Increased muscle oxidative potential following resistance training induced fibre hypertrophy in young men.* Appl Physiol Nutr Metab, 2006. **31**(5): p. 495-501.

57. Sugie, M., et al., *Relationship between skeletal muscle mass and cardiac function during exercise in community-dwelling older adults.* ESC Heart Fail, 2017. **4**(4): p. 409-416.

58. Medicine, A.A.C.o.S. *High-Intensity Interval Training.* 2014 [cited 2021 3/11/2021]; Available from: https://www.acsm.org/docs/default-source/files-for-resource-library/high-intensity-interval-training.pdf.

59. Ito, S., *High-intensity interval training for health benefits and care of cardiac diseases - The key to an efficient exercise protocol.* World J Cardiol, 2019. **11**(7): p. 171-188.

60. Ramos, J.S., et al., *The impact of high-intensity interval training versus moderate-intensity continuous training on vascular function: a systematic review and meta-analysis.* Sports Med, 2015. **45**(5): p. 679-92.

61. Weston, K.S., U. Wisløff, and J.S. Coombes, *High-intensity interval training in patients with lifestyle-induced cardiometabolic disease: a systematic review and meta-analysis.* Br J Sports Med, 2014. **48**(16): p. 1227-34.

62. Callahan, M.J., et al., *Can High-Intensity Interval Training Promote Skeletal Muscle Anabolism?* Sports Med, 2021. **51**(3): p. 405-421.

63. Scalzo, R.L., et al., *Greater muscle protein synthesis and mitochondrial biogenesis in males compared with females during sprint interval training.* Faseb j, 2014. **28**(6): p. 2705-14.

64. Martinez-Valdes, E., et al., *Differential Motor Unit Changes after Endurance or High-Intensity Interval Training.* Med Sci Sports Exerc, 2017. **49**(6): p. 1126-1136.

65. García-Pinillos, F., et al., *A High Intensity Interval Training (HIIT)-Based Running Plan Improves Athletic Performance by Improving Muscle Power.* J Strength Cond Res, 2017. **31**(1): p. 146-153.

66. Konopka, A.R. and M.P. Harber, *Skeletal muscle hypertrophy after aerobic exercise training.* Exerc Sport Sci Rev, 2014. **42**(2): p. 53-61.

67. Di Donato, D.M., et al., *Influence of aerobic exercise intensity on myofibrillar and mitochondrial protein synthesis in young men during early and late postexercise recovery.* Am J Physiol Endocrinol Metab, 2014. **306**(9): p. E1025-32.

68. Grgic, J., et al., *Does Aerobic Training Promote the Same Skeletal Muscle Hypertrophy as Resistance Training? A Systematic Review and Meta-Analysis.* Sports Medicine, 2019. **49**(2): p. 233-254.

69. Wilkinson, S.B., et al., *Differential effects of resistance and endurance exercise in the fed state on signalling molecule phosphorylation and protein synthesis in human muscle.* J Physiol, 2008. **586**(15): p. 3701-17.

70. Anton, S.D., et al., *Flipping the Metabolic Switch: Understanding and Applying the Health Benefits of Fasting.* Obesity (Silver Spring), 2018. **26**(2): p. 254-268.

Chapter 8

1. Elisia, I. and G. Krystal, *The Pros and Cons of Low Carbohydrate and Ketogenic Diets in the Prevention and Treatment of Cancer.* Front Nutr, 2021. **8**: p. 634845.

2. Szypowska, A. and B. Regulska-Ilow, *Significance of low-carbohydrate diets and fasting in patients with cancer.* Rocz Panstw Zakl Hig, 2019. **70**(4): p. 325-336.

3. Włodarek, D., *Role of Ketogenic Diets in Neurodegenerative Diseases (Alzheimer's Disease and Parkinson's Disease).* Nutrients, 2019. **11**(1).

4. Liumbruno, G.M., *Proteomics: applications in transfusion medicine.* Blood Transfus, 2008. **6**(2): p. 70-85.

5. Martens, E.A., S.G. Lemmens, and M.S. Westerterp-Plantenga, *Protein leverage affects energy intake of high-protein diets in humans.* Am J Clin Nutr, 2013. **97**(1): p. 86-93.

6. Gosby, A.K., et al., *Testing protein leverage in lean humans: a randomised controlled experimental study.* PLoS One, 2011. **6**(10): p. e25929.

7. Austin, G.L., L.G. Ogden, and J.O. Hill, *Trends in carbohydrate, fat, and protein intakes and association with energy intake in normal-weight, overweight, and obese individuals: 1971-2006.* Am J Clin Nutr, 2011. **93**(4): p. 836-43.

8. Simpson, S.J. and D. Raubenheimer, *Obesity: the protein leverage hypothesis.* Obes Rev, 2005. **6**(2): p. 133-42.

9. Colagiuri, S. and J. Brand Miller, *The 'carnivore connection'--evolutionary aspects of insulin resistance.* Eur J Clin Nutr, 2002. **56 Suppl 1**: p. S30-5.

10. Brand-Miller, J.C., H.J. Griffin, and S. Colagiuri, *The carnivore connection hypothesis: revisited.* J Obes, 2012. **2012**: p. 258624.

11. Kirwan, R.P., et al., *Protein interventions augment the effect of resistance exercise on appendicular lean mass and handgrip strength in older adults: a systematic review and meta-analysis of randomized controlled trials.* The American Journal of Clinical Nutrition, 2021.

12. Jun, S., et al., *Dietary Protein Intake Is Positively Associated with Appendicular Lean Mass and Handgrip Strength among Middle-Aged US Adults.* The Journal of Nutrition, 2021. **151**(12): p. 3755-3763.

13. Wu, G., *Dietary protein intake and human health.* Food Funct, 2016. **7**(3): p. 1251-65.

14. Wu, G., F.W. Bazer, and H.R. Cross, *Land-based production of animal protein: impacts, efficiency, and sustainability.* Ann N Y Acad Sci, 2014. **1328**: p. 18-28.

15. Willcox, D.C., G. Scapagnini, and B.J. Willcox, *Healthy aging diets other than the Mediterranean: a focus on the Okinawan diet.* Mech Ageing Dev, 2014. **136-137**: p. 148-62.

16. Provenza, F.D., S.L. Kronberg, and P. Gregorini, *Is Grassfed Meat and Dairy Better for Human and Environmental Health?* Front Nutr, 2019. **6**: p. 26.

17. Crittenden, A.N. and D.A. Zes, *Food Sharing among Hadza Hunter-Gatherer Children.* PLoS One, 2015. **10**(7): p. e0131996.

18. Levine, M.E., et al., *Low protein intake is associated with a major reduction in IGF-1, cancer, and overall mortality in the 65 and younger but not older population.* Cell Metab, 2014. **19**(3): p. 407-17.

19. Norton, L. *Protein experts respond to recent anti-protein claims.* 2014 [cited 2021 06/08/2021].

20. Mora-Bermúdez, F., et al., *Differences and similarities between human and chimpanzee neural progenitors during cerebral cortex development.* Elife, 2016. **5**.

21. Milton, K., *The critical role played by animal source foods in human (Homo) evolution.* J Nutr, 2003. **133**(11 Suppl 2): p. 3886s-3892s.

22. Mackie, R.I., *Mutualistic fermentative digestion in the gastrointestinal tract: diversity and evolution.* Integr Comp Biol, 2002. **42**(2): p. 319-26.

23. Hahn, K.E., et al., *Impact of Arachidonic and Docosahexaenoic Acid Supplementation on Neural and Immune Development in the Young Pig.* Frontiers in Nutrition, 2020. **7**(214).

24. Cordain, L., B.A. Watkins, and N.J. Mann, *Fatty acid composition and energy density of foods available to African hominids. Evolutionary implications for human brain development.* World Rev Nutr Diet, 2001. **90**: p. 144-61.

25. Venkatramanan, S., et al., *Vitamin B-12 and Cognition in Children.* Adv Nutr, 2016. **7**(5): p. 879-88.

26. Watanabe, F., et al., *Pseudovitamin B(12) is the predominant cobamide of an algal health food, spirulina tablets.* J Agric Food Chem, 1999. **47**(11): p. 4736-41.

27. Vogiatzoglou, A., et al., *Vitamin B12 status and rate of brain volume loss in community-dwelling elderly.* Neurology, 2008. **71**(11): p. 826-32.

28. Hawks, J., *How has the human brain evolved?*, in *Scientific American Mind.* 2013.

29. Prasad, A.S., *Discovery of human zinc deficiency: its impact on human health and disease.* Adv Nutr, 2013. **4**(2): p. 176-90.

30. Gower-Winter, S.D. and C.W. Levenson, *Zinc in the central nervous system: From molecules to behavior.* Biofactors, 2012. **38**(3): p. 186-93.

31. Maares, M. and H. Haase, *A Guide to Human Zinc Absorption: General Overview and Recent Advances of In Vitro Intestinal Models.* Nutrients, 2020. **12**(3).

32. Foster, M., et al., *Effect of vegetarian diets on zinc status: a systematic review and meta-analysis of studies in humans.* J Sci Food Agric, 2013. **93**(10): p. 2362-71.

33. Derbyshire, E., *Could we be overlooking a potential choline crisis in the United Kingdom?* BMJ Nutrition, Prevention & Health, 2019. 2: p. bmjnph-2019.

34. Smith, S.B., *Marbling and Its Nutritional Impact on Risk Factors for Cardiovascular Disease.* Korean J Food Sci Anim Resour, 2016. **36**(4): p. 435-44.

35. DiNicolantonio, J.J. and J.H. O'Keefe, *Effects of dietary fats on blood lipids: a review of direct comparison trials.* Open Heart, 2018. **5**(2): p. e000871.

36. Caldas, A.P.S., et al., *Dietary fatty acids as nutritional modulators of sirtuins: a systematic review.* Nutr Rev, 2021. **79**(2): p. 235-246.

37. Teles, F.F., *Chronic poisoning by hydrogen cyanide in cassava and its prevention in Africa and Latin America.* Food Nutr Bull, 2002. **23**(4): p. 407-12.

38. Gurm, H.S. and M.S. Lauer, *Predicting incidence of some critical events by sun signs—the Pisces study.* ACC Current Journal Review, 2003. **12**(1): p. 22-24.

39. Marks, G.C., M.C. Hughes, and J.C. van der Pols, *Relative validity of food intake estimates using a food frequency questionnaire is associated with sex, age, and other personal characteristics.* J Nutr, 2006. **136**(2): p. 459-65.

40. Schwingshackl, L., et al., *Food groups and risk of all-cause mortality: a systematic review and meta-analysis of prospective studies.* Am J Clin Nutr, 2017. **105**(6): p. 1462-1473.

41. Ioannidis, J.P.A., *The Challenge of Reforming Nutritional Epidemiologic Research.* Jama, 2018. **320**(10): p. 969-970.

42. Agriculture, U.D.o.H.a.H.S.a.U.D.o., *2015-2020 Dietary Guidelines for Americans*, U.a. HHS, Editor. 2015.

43. Bouvard, V., et al., *Carcinogenicity of consumption of red and processed meat.* Lancet Oncol, 2015. **16**(16): p. 1599-600.

44. Hur, S.J., et al., *Controversy on the correlation of red and processed meat consumption with colorectal cancer risk: an Asian perspective.* Crit Rev Food Sci Nutr, 2019. **59**(21): p. 3526-3537.

45. *Unprocessed Red Meat and Processed Meat Consumption: Dietary Guideline Recommendations From the Nutritional Recommendations (NutriRECS) Consortium.* Annals of Internal Medicine, 2019. **171**(10): p. 756-764.

46. Astrup, A., et al., *Saturated Fats and Health: A Reassessment and Proposal for Food-Based Recommendations: JACC State-of-the-Art Review.* J Am Coll Cardiol, 2020. **76**(7): p. 844-857.

47. Dehghan, M., et al., *Associations of fats and carbohydrate intake with cardiovascular disease and mortality in 18 countries from five continents (PURE): a prospective cohort study.* Lancet, 2017. **390**(10107): p. 2050-2062.

48. Mente, A., et al., *Association of dietary nutrients with blood lipids and blood pressure in 18 countries: a cross-sectional analysis from the PURE study.* Lancet Diabetes Endocrinol, 2017. **5**(10): p. 774-787.

49. Micha, R., S.K. Wallace, and D. Mozaffarian, *Red and processed meat consumption and risk of incident coronary heart disease, stroke, and diabetes mellitus: a systematic review and meta-analysis.* Circulation, 2010. **121**(21): p. 2271-83.

50. Ben-Dor, M., R. Sirtoli, and R. Barkai, *The evolution of the human trophic level during the Pleistocene.* Am J Phys Anthropol, 2021. **175 Suppl 72**: p. 27-56.

51. Wu, G., et al., *Composition of free and peptide-bound amino acids in beef chuck, loin, and round cuts1,2.* Journal of Animal Science, 2016. **94**(6): p. 2603-2613.

52. Fannin, B., *U.S. decline in meat protein consumption raises concern for Texas A&M scientist.*, in *AgriLife Today.* 2016.

53. Konstantinidi, M. and A.E. Koutelidakis, *Functional Foods and Bioactive Compounds: A Review of Its Possible Role on Weight*

Management and Obesity's Metabolic Consequences. Medicines (Basel), 2019. **6**(3).

54. Wu, G., *Important roles of dietary taurine, creatine, carnosine, anserine and 4-hydroxyproline in human nutrition and health.* Amino Acids, 2020. **52**(3): p. 329-360.

55. Glatzle, A., *Questioning key conclusions of FAO publications 'Livestock's Long Shadow' (2006) appearing again in 'Tackling Climate Change Through Livestock' (2013).* Pastoralism, 2014. **4**(1): p. 1.

56. Pitesky, M.E., K.R. Stackhouse, and F.M. Mitloehner, *Chapter 1 - Clearing the Air: Livestock's Contribution to Climate Change*, in *Advances in Agronomy*, D.L. Sparks, Editor. 2009, Academic Press. p. 1-40.

57. Raiten, D.J., et al., *Understanding the Intersection of Climate/Environmental Change, Health, Agriculture, and Improved Nutrition: A Case Study on Micronutrient Nutrition and Animal Source Foods.* Curr Dev Nutr, 2020. **4**(7): p. nzaa087.

58. Rasmussen, C., *NASA-led study solves a methane puzzle*, in *Jet Propulsion Laboratory News*. 2018, California Institute of Technology: California.

59. Programme, J.F.I., *Belching ruminants, a minor player in atmosphereic methane.* 2008: Vienna, Austria.

60. Stanley, P.L., et al., *Impacts of soil carbon sequestration on life cycle greenhouse gas emissions in Midwestern USA beef finishing systems.* Agricultural Systems, 2018. **162**: p. 249-258.

61. Viglizzo, E.F., et al., *Reassessing the role of grazing lands in carbon-balance estimations: Meta-analysis and review.* Sci Total Environ, 2019. **661**: p. 531-542.

62. White, R.R. and M.B. Hall, *Nutritional and greenhouse gas impacts of removing animals from US agriculture.* Proc Natl Acad Sci U S A, 2017. **114**(48): p. E10301-e10308.

63. Agency, U.S.E.P. *Inventory of U.S. greenhouse gas emmissions and sinks.* 2019 [cited 2021 5/18/2021]; Available from: https://www.epa.gov/ghgemissions/inventory-us-greenhouse-gas-emissions-and-sinks.

64. Canada, D.F.o. *We Cannot Eat Our Way Out of Climate Change, Says Expert.* [communications] 2019 2019 [cited 2021 10/1/2021]; Available from: https://dairyfarmersofcanada.ca/en/we-cannot-eat-our-way-out-climate-change-says-expert.

65. Layman, D.K., *Assessing the Role of Cattle in Sustainable Food Systems.* Nutrition Today, 2018. **53**(4): p. 160-165.

66. Rehkamp, S. *A Look at calorie sources in the American Diet.* 2016 12/5/2016 [cited 2022 2/25/22]; Available from: https://www.ers.usda.gov/amber-waves/2016/december/a-look-at-calorie-sources-in-the-american-diet/.

67. van Vliet, S., et al., *A metabolomics comparison of plant-based meat and grass-fed meat indicates large nutritional differences despite comparable Nutrition Facts panels.* Sci Rep, 2021. **11**(1): p. 13828.

68. Escrich, R., et al., *A high-corn-oil diet strongly stimulates mammary carcinogenesis, while a high-extra-virgin-olive-oil diet has a weak effect, through changes in metabolism, immune system function and proliferation/apoptosis pathways.* The Journal of Nutritional Biochemistry, 2019. **64**: p. 218-227.

69. Williams, K.A., Sr., et al., *The 2015 Dietary Guidelines Advisory Committee Report Concerning Dietary Cholesterol.* Am J Cardiol, 2015. **116**(9): p. 1479-80.

70. Lin, H.P., et al., *Dietary Cholesterol, Lipid Levels, and Cardiovascular Risk among Adults with Diabetes or Impaired Fasting Glucose in the Framingham Offspring Study.* Nutrients, 2018. **10**(6).

71. Nimni, M.E., B. Han, and F. Cordoba, *Are we getting enough sulfur in our diet?* Nutrition & Metabolism, 2007. **4**(1): p. 24.

72. Chung, H.Y., H.M. Rasmussen, and E.J. Johnson, *Lutein bioavailability is higher from lutein-enriched eggs than from supplements and spinach in men.* J Nutr, 2004. **134**(8): p. 1887-93.

73. Ulven, S.M., et al., *Milk and Dairy Product Consumption and Inflammatory Biomarkers: An Updated Systematic Review of Randomized Clinical Trials.* Adv Nutr, 2019. **10**(suppl_2): p. S239-s250.

74. Labonté, M., et al., *Impact of dairy products on biomarkers of inflammation: a systematic review of randomized controlled*

nutritional intervention studies in overweight and obese adults. Am J Clin Nutr, 2013. **97**(4): p. 706-17.

75. Bordoni, A., et al., *Dairy products and inflammation: A review of the clinical evidence.* Crit Rev Food Sci Nutr, 2017. **57**(12): p. 2497-2525.

76. Mozaffarian, D., *Dairy foods, dairy fat, diabetes, and death: what can be learned from 3 large new investigations?* Am J Clin Nutr, 2019. **110**(5): p. 1053-1054.

77. Ho, H.J., M. Komai, and H. Shirakawa, *Beneficial Effects of Vitamin K Status on Glycemic Regulation and Diabetes Mellitus: A Mini-Review.* Nutrients, 2020. **12**(8).

78. Nguyen, D.D., et al., *Formation and Degradation of Beta-casomorphins in Dairy Processing.* Crit Rev Food Sci Nutr, 2015. **55**(14): p. 1955-67.

79. Zhang, W., et al., *The protective effects of beta-casomorphin-7 against glucose -induced renal oxidative stress in vivo and vitro.* PLoS One, 2013. **8**(5): p. e63472.

80. Zhang, Z., et al., β-Casomorphin-7 Ameliorates Sepsis-Induced Acute Kidney Injury by Targeting NF-κB Pathway. Med Sci Monit, 2019. **25**: p. 121-127.

81. De Noni I, F.R., Korhonen HJT, et al. , *Review of the potantial health impact of beat-casomorphins and related peptides.* EFSA Scientific Report, 2009. **231**: p. 1-107.

82. Asledottir, T., et al., *Degradation of β-casomorphin-7 through in vitro gastrointestinal and jejunal brush border membrane digestion.* J Dairy Sci, 2019. **102**(10): p. 8622-8629.

83. Gupta, R.S., et al., *Prevalence and Severity of Food Allergies Among US Adults.* JAMA Netw Open, 2019. **2**(1): p. e185630.

84. Fontana, L., et al., *Dietary protein restriction inhibits tumor growth in human xenograft models.* Oncotarget, 2013. **4**(12): p. 2451-61.

85. Papadopoli, D., et al., *mTOR as a central regulator of lifespan and aging.* F1000Res, 2019. **8**.

86. Kitada, M., et al., *The impact of dietary protein intake on longevity and metabolic health.* EBioMedicine, 2019. **43**: p. 632-640.

87. Gui, Y.S., et al., *mTOR Overactivation and Compromised Autophagy in the Pathogenesis of Pulmonary Fibrosis*. PLoS One, 2015. **10**(9): p. e0138625.

88. Yoon, M.S., *The Role of Mammalian Target of Rapamycin (mTOR) in Insulin Signaling*. Nutrients, 2017. **9**(11).

89. Gran, P. and D. Cameron-Smith, *The actions of exogenous leucine on mTOR signalling and amino acid transporters in human myotubes*. BMC Physiol, 2011. **11**: p. 10.

90. Sangüesa, G., et al., *mTOR is a Key Protein Involved in the Metabolic Effects of Simple Sugars*. Int J Mol Sci, 2019. **20**(5).

91. D'Hulst, G., E. Masschelein, and K. De Bock, *Dampened Muscle mTORC1 Response Following Ingestion of High-Quality Plant-Based Protein and Insect Protein Compared to Whey*. Nutrients, 2021. **13**(5).

92. Hever, J. and R.J. Cronise, *Plant-based nutrition for healthcare professionals: implementing diet as a primary modality in the prevention and treatment of chronic disease*. J Geriatr Cardiol, 2017. **14**(5): p. 355-368.

93. van Vliet, S., N.A. Burd, and L.J. van Loon, *The Skeletal Muscle Anabolic Response to Plant- versus Animal-Based Protein Consumption*. J Nutr, 2015. **145**(9): p. 1981-91.

94. Huang, M. and J.W. Joseph, *Assessment of the Metabolic Pathways Associated With Glucose-Stimulated Biphasic Insulin Secretion*. Endocrinology, 2014. **155**(5): p. 1653-1666.

95. Devkota, S. and D.K. Layman, *Increased ratio of dietary carbohydrate to protein shifts the focus of metabolic signaling from skeletal muscle to adipose*. Nutr Metab (Lond), 2011. **8**(1): p. 13.

96. López Teros, M.T., C.F. Ramírez, and H. Alemán-Mateo, *Hyperinsulinemia is associated with the loss of appendicular skeletal muscle mass at 4.6 year follow-up in older men and women*. Clin Nutr, 2015. **34**(5): p. 931-6.

97. Lasker, D.A., E.M. Evans, and D.K. Layman, *Moderate carbohydrate, moderate protein weight loss diet reduces cardiovascular disease risk compared to high carbohydrate, low protein diet in obese adults: A randomized clinical trial*. Nutr Metab (Lond), 2008. **5**: p. 30.

98. Phinney, J.S.V.a.S.D., *The Art and Science of Low Carbohydrate Living.* 2011: Beyond Obesity LLC. 316.

99. Hallberg, S.J., et al., *Effectiveness and Safety of a Novel Care Model for the Management of Type 2 Diabetes at 1 Year: An Open-Label, Non-Randomized, Controlled Study.* Diabetes Ther, 2018. **9**(2): p. 583-612.

100. Volek, J.S. and S.D. Phinney, *The Art and Science of Low Carbohydrate Performance: A Revolutionary Program to Extend Your Physical and Mental Performance Envelope.* 2012: Beyond Obesity LLC.

101. Young, C.M., et al., *Effect of body composition and other parameters in obese young men of carbohydrate level of reduction diet.* Am J Clin Nutr, 1971. **24**(3): p. 290-6.

102. Wallace, M.A., et al., *The ketogenic diet preserves skeletal muscle with aging in mice.* Aging Cell, 2021. **20**(4): p. e13322.

103. Nair, K.S., et al., *Effect of beta-hydroxybutyrate on whole-body leucine kinetics and fractional mixed skeletal muscle protein synthesis in humans.* J Clin Invest, 1988. **82**(1): p. 198-205.

104. Vandoorne, T., et al., *Intake of a Ketone Ester Drink during Recovery from Exercise Promotes mTORC1 Signaling but Not Glycogen Resynthesis in Human Muscle.* Front Physiol, 2017. **8**: p. 310.

105. Wilson, J.M., et al., *Effects of Ketogenic Dieting on Body Composition, Strength, Power, and Hormonal Profiles in Resistance Training Men.* J Strength Cond Res, 2020. **34**(12): p. 3463-3474.

106. Volek, J.S., et al., *Body composition and hormonal responses to a carbohydrate-restricted diet.* Metabolism, 2002. **51**(7): p. 864-70.

107. Paoli, A., et al., *Ketogenic diet does not affect strength performance in elite artistic gymnasts.* J Int Soc Sports Nutr, 2012. **9**(1): p. 34.

108. Gregory RM, e.a., *A low-carbohydrate ketogenic diet combined with 6-weeks of crossfit training improves body composition and performance.* Int J Sports Exerc Med, 2017. **3**(2): p. 1-10.

109. Rafiullah, M., M. Musambil, and S.K. David, *Effect of a very low-carbohydrate ketogenic diet vs recommended diets in patients with type 2 diabetes: a meta-analysis.* Nutrition Reviews, 2021.

Chapter 9

1. Mattson, M.P., V.D. Longo, and M. Harvie, *Impact of intermittent fasting on health and disease processes.* Ageing Res Rev, 2017. **39**: p. 46-58.

2. Longo, V.D. and M.P. Mattson, *Fasting: molecular mechanisms and clinical applications.* Cell Metab, 2014. **19**(2): p. 181-92.

3. Patterson, R.E., et al., *Intermittent Fasting and Human Metabolic Health.* J Acad Nutr Diet, 2015. **115**(8): p. 1203-12.

4. Okada, C., et al., *The Association of Having a Late Dinner or Bedtime Snack and Skipping Breakfast with Overweight in Japanese Women.* J Obes, 2019. **2019**: p. 2439571.

5. Yoshida, J., et al., *Association of night eating habits with metabolic syndrome and its components: a longitudinal study.* BMC Public Health, 2018. **18**(1): p. 1366.

6. Stokes, T., et al., *Recent Perspectives Regarding the Role of Dietary Protein for the Promotion of Muscle Hypertrophy with Resistance Exercise Training.* Nutrients, 2018. **10**(2).

7. de Cabo, R. and M.P. Mattson, *Effects of Intermittent Fasting on Health, Aging, and Disease.* N Engl J Med, 2019. **381**(26): p. 2541-2551.

8. Phillips, M.C.L., *Fasting as a Therapy in Neurological Disease.* Nutrients, 2019. **11**(10).

9. Zimmermann, A., et al., *When less is more: hormesis against stress and disease.* Microb Cell, 2014. **1**(5): p. 150-153.

10. Lee, J., et al., *Adaptive cellular stress pathways as therapeutic targets of dietary phytochemicals: focus on the nervous system.* Pharmacol Rev, 2014. **66**(3): p. 815-68.

11. Anton, S.D., et al., *Flipping the Metabolic Switch: Understanding and Applying the Health Benefits of Fasting.* Obesity (Silver Spring), 2018. **26**(2): p. 254-268.

12. Freese, J., et al., *The sedentary (r)evolution: Have we lost our metabolic flexibility?* F1000Res, 2017. **6**: p. 1787.

13. Grajower, M.M. and B.D. Horne, *Clinical Management of Intermittent Fasting in Patients with Diabetes Mellitus.* Nutrients, 2019. **11**(4).

14. Wang, A., et al., *Opposing Effects of Fasting Metabolism on Tissue Tolerance in Bacterial and Viral Inflammation.* Cell, 2016. **166**(6): p. 1512-1525.e12.

15. Moro, T., et al., *Effects of eight weeks of time-restricted feeding (16/8) on basal metabolism, maximal strength, body composition, inflammation, and cardiovascular risk factors in resistance-trained males.* J Transl Med, 2016. **14**(1): p. 290.

16. Bhutani, S., et al., *Alternate day fasting and endurance exercise combine to reduce body weight and favorably alter plasma lipids in obese humans.* Obesity (Silver Spring), 2013. **21**(7): p. 1370-9.

17. Lowe, D.A., et al., *Effects of Time-Restricted Eating on Weight Loss and Other Metabolic Parameters in Women and Men With Overweight and Obesity: The TREAT Randomized Clinical Trial.* JAMA Intern Med, 2020. **180**(11): p. 1491-1499.

18. Tinsley, G.M., et al., *Time-restricted feeding in young men performing resistance training: A randomized controlled trial.* Eur J Sport Sci, 2017. **17**(2): p. 200-207.

19. Soenen, S., et al., *Normal protein intake is required for body weight loss and weight maintenance, and elevated protein intake for additional preservation of resting energy expenditure and fat free mass.* J Nutr, 2013. **143**(5): p. 591-6.

20. Martinez-Lopez, N., et al., *System-wide Benefits of Intermeal Fasting by Autophagy.* Cell Metab, 2017. **26**(6): p. 856-871.e5.

21. Park, S.S., Y.K. Seo, and K.S. Kwon, *Sarcopenia targeting with autophagy mechanism by exercise.* BMB Rep, 2019. **52**(1): p. 64-69.

22. Madreiter-Sokolowski, C.T., et al., *Targeting Mitochondria to Counteract Age-Related Cellular Dysfunction.* Genes (Basel), 2018. **9**(3).

23. Vendelbo, M.H., et al., *Exercise and fasting activate growth hormone-dependent myocellular signal transducer and activator of transcription-5b phosphorylation and insulin-like growth factor-I messenger ribonucleic acid expression in humans.* J Clin Endocrinol Metab, 2010. **95**(9): p. E64-8.

24. Møller, N. and J.O.L. Jørgensen, *Effects of Growth Hormone on Glucose, Lipid, and Protein Metabolism in Human Subjects.* Endocrine Reviews, 2009. **30**(2): p. 152-177.

Chapter 10

1. Devries, M. and S. Phillips, *Supplemental Protein in Support of Muscle Mass and Health: Advantage Whey.* Journal of Food Science, 2015. **80**.

2. Phillips, S.M., D. Paddon-Jones, and D.K. Layman, *Optimizing Adult Protein Intake During Catabolic Health Conditions.* Adv Nutr, 2020. **11**(4): p. S1058-s1069.

3. Farup, J., et al., *Whey protein supplementation accelerates satellite cell proliferation during recovery from eccentric exercise.* Amino Acids, 2014. **46**(11): p. 2503-16.

4. Arentson-Lantz, E.J., et al., *Improving Dietary Protein Quality Reduces the Negative Effects of Physical Inactivity on Body Composition and Muscle Function.* J Gerontol A Biol Sci Med Sci, 2019. **74**(10): p. 1605-1611.

5. Pal, S. and V. Ellis, *The acute effects of four protein meals on insulin, glucose, appetite and energy intake in lean men.* Br J Nutr, 2010. **104**(8): p. 1241-8.

6. Miller, P.E., D.D. Alexander, and V. Perez, *Effects of whey protein and resistance exercise on body composition: a meta-analysis of randomized controlled trials.* J Am Coll Nutr, 2014. **33**(2): p. 163-75.

7. Jakubowicz, D., et al., *Incretin, insulinotropic and glucose-lowering effects of whey protein pre-load in type 2 diabetes: a randomised clinical trial.* Diabetologia, 2014. **57**(9): p. 1807-11.

8. Madonna, R. and R. De Caterina, *Atherogenesis and diabetes: focus on insulin resistance and hyperinsulinemia.* Rev Esp Cardiol (Engl Ed), 2012. **65**(4): p. 309-13.

9. Pal, S., V. Ellis, and S. Dhaliwal, *Effects of whey protein isolate on body composition, lipids, insulin and glucose in overweight and obese individuals.* British Journal of Nutrition, 2010. **104**(5): p. 716-723.

10. Fouré, A. and D. Bendahan, *Is Branched-Chain Amino Acids Supplementation an Efficient Nutritional Strategy to Alleviate Skeletal Muscle Damage? A Systematic Review.* Nutrients, 2017. **9**(10).

11. Moberg, M., et al., *Activation of mTORC1 by leucine is potentiated by branched-chain amino acids and even more so by essential amino acids following resistance exercise.* Am J Physiol Cell Physiol, 2016. **310**(11): p. C874-84.

12. Santos, C.S. and F.E.L. Nascimento, *Isolated branched-chain amino acid intake and muscle protein synthesis in humans: a biochemical review.* Einstein (Sao Paulo), 2019. **17**(3): p. eRB4898.

13. Jackman, S.R., et al., *Branched-Chain Amino Acid Ingestion Stimulates Muscle Myofibrillar Protein Synthesis following Resistance Exercise in Humans.* Frontiers in Physiology, 2017. **8**(390).

14. Churchward-Venne, T.A., et al., *Leucine supplementation of a low-protein mixed macronutrient beverage enhances myofibrillar protein synthesis in young men: a double-blind, randomized trial.* Am J Clin Nutr, 2014. **99**(2): p. 276-86.

15. McKendry, J., et al., *Nutritional Supplements to Support Resistance Exercise in Countering the Sarcopenia of Aging.* Nutrients, 2020. **12**(7).

16. Morton, R., et al., *Defining anabolic resistance: Implications for delivery of clinical care nutrition.* Current Opinion in Critical Care, 2018. **24**: p. 1.

17. Osmond, A.D., et al., *The Effects of Leucine-Enriched Branched-Chain Amino Acid Supplementation on Recovery After High-Intensity Resistance Exercise.* Int J Sports Physiol Perform, 2019. **14**(8): p. 1081-1088.

18. Chazaud, B., *Inflammation and Skeletal Muscle Regeneration: Leave It to the Macrophages!* Trends in Immunology, 2020. **41**(6): p. 481-492.

19. Khemtong, C., et al., *Does Branched-Chain Amino Acids (BCAAs) Supplementation Attenuate Muscle Damage Markers and Soreness after Resistance Exercise in Trained Males? A Meta-Analysis of Randomized Controlled Trials.* Nutrients, 2021. **13**(6).

20. Rahimlou, M., et al., *Reduction of Muscle Injuries and Improved Post-exercise Recovery by Branched-Chain Amino Acid Supplementation: A Systematic Review and Meta-Analysis.* Journal of Nutrition,Fasting and Health, 2020. **8**(1): p. 1-16.

21. Gee, T.I. and S. Deniel, *Branched-chain aminoacid supplementation attenuates a decrease in power-producing ability following acute strength training.* J Sports Med Phys Fitness, 2016. **56**(12): p. 1511-1517.

22. Kim, D.H., et al., *Effect of BCAA intake during endurance exercises on fatigue substances, muscle damage substances, and energy metabolism substances.* J Exerc Nutrition Biochem, 2013. **17**(4): p. 169-80.

23. Manaf, F.A., et al., *Branched-chain amino acid supplementation improves cycling performance in untrained cyclists.* J Sci Med Sport, 2021. **24**(4): p. 412-417.

24. Wu, G., *Important roles of dietary taurine, creatine, carnosine, anserine and 4-hydroxyproline in human nutrition and health.* Amino Acids, 2020. **52**(3): p. 329-360.

25. Smith, R.N., A.S. Agharkar, and E.B. Gonzales, *A review of creatine supplementation in age-related diseases: more than a supplement for athletes.* F1000Res, 2014. **3**: p. 222.

26. Candow, D.G., et al., *Effectiveness of Creatine Supplementation on Aging Muscle and Bone: Focus on Falls Prevention and Inflammation.* J Clin Med, 2019. **8**(4).

27. Wallimann, T., M. Tokarska-Schlattner, and U. Schlattner, *The creatine kinase system and pleiotropic effects of creatine.* Amino Acids, 2011. **40**(5): p. 1271-96.

28. Farshidfar, F., M.A. Pinder, and S.B. Myrie, *Creatine Supplementation and Skeletal Muscle Metabolism for Building Muscle Mass- Review of the Potential Mechanisms of Action.* Curr Protein Pept Sci, 2017. **18**(12): p. 1273-1287.

29. Chilibeck, P.D., et al., *Effect of creatine supplementation during resistance training on lean tissue mass and muscular strength in older adults: a meta-analysis.* Open Access J Sports Med, 2017. **8**: p. 213-226.

30. Kreider, R.B., et al., *International Society of Sports Nutrition position stand: safety and efficacy of creatine supplementation in exercise, sport, and medicine.* J Int Soc Sports Nutr, 2017. **14**: p. 18.

31. Gao, H., et al., *Fish oil supplementation and insulin sensitivity: a systematic review and meta-analysis.* Lipids Health Dis, 2017. **16**(1): p. 131.

32. Bernasconi, A.A., et al., *Effect of Omega-3 Dosage on Cardiovascular Outcomes: An Updated Meta-Analysis and Meta-Regression of Interventional Trials.* Mayo Clin Proc, 2021. **96**(2): p. 304-313.

33. Canhada, S., et al., *Omega-3 fatty acids' supplementation in Alzheimer's disease: A systematic review.* Nutr Neurosci, 2018. **21**(8): p. 529-538.

34. Wan, Y., et al., *Fish, long chain omega-3 polyunsaturated fatty acids consumption, and risk of all-cause mortality: a systematic review and dose-response meta-analysis from 23 independent prospective cohort studies.* Asia Pac J Clin Nutr, 2017. **26**(5): p. 939-956.

35. Gerling, C.J., et al., *Incorporation of Omega-3 Fatty Acids Into Human Skeletal Muscle Sarcolemmal and Mitochondrial Membranes Following 12 Weeks of Fish Oil Supplementation.* Frontiers in Physiology, 2019. **10**(348).

36. Smith, G.I., et al., *Omega-3 polyunsaturated fatty acids augment the muscle protein anabolic response to hyperinsulinaemia-hyperaminoacidaemia in healthy young and middle-aged men and women.* Clin Sci (Lond), 2011. **121**(6): p. 267-78.

37. Smith, G.I., et al., *Dietary omega-3 fatty acid supplementation increases the rate of muscle protein synthesis in older adults: a randomized controlled trial.* Am J Clin Nutr, 2011. **93**(2): p. 402-12.

38. Lalia, A.Z., et al., *Influence of omega-3 fatty acids on skeletal muscle protein metabolism and mitochondrial bioenergetics in older adults.* Aging, 2017. **9**(4): p. 1096-1129.

39. Rodacki, C.L., et al., *Fish-oil supplementation enhances the effects of strength training in elderly women.* Am J Clin Nutr, 2012. **95**(2): p. 428-36.

40. Smith, G.I., et al., *Fish oil–derived n–3 PUFA therapy increases muscle mass and function in healthy older adults1.* The American Journal of Clinical Nutrition, 2015. **102**(1): p. 115-122.

41. Mcglory, C., et al., *Omega-3 fatty acid supplementation attenuates skeletal muscle disuse atrophy during two weeks of unilateral leg immobilization in healthy young women.* The FASEB Journal, 2019. **33**(3): p. 4586-4597.

42. Montenegro, K.R., et al., *Mechanisms of vitamin D action in skeletal muscle.* Nutr Res Rev, 2019. **32**(2): p. 192-204.

43. Garcia, L.A., et al., *1,25(OH)2vitamin D3 stimulates myogenic differentiation by inhibiting cell proliferation and modulating the expression of promyogenic growth factors and myostatin in C2C12 skeletal muscle cells.* Endocrinology, 2011. **152**(8): p. 2976-86.

44. van der Meijden, K., et al., *Effects of 1,25(OH)2 D3 and 25(OH) D3 on C2C12 Myoblast Proliferation, Differentiation, and Myotube Hypertrophy.* J Cell Physiol, 2016. **231**(11): p. 2517-28.

45. Owens, D.J., et al., *A systems-based investigation into vitamin D and skeletal muscle repair, regeneration, and hypertrophy.* Am J Physiol Endocrinol Metab, 2015. **309**(12): p. E1019-31.

46. Antoniak, A.E. and C.A. Greig, *The effect of combined resistance exercise training and vitamin D_3 supplementation on musculoskeletal health and function in older adults: a systematic review and meta-analysis.* BMJ Open, 2017. 7(7): p. e014619.

47. Dahlquist, D.T., B.P. Dieter, and M.S. Koehle, *Plausible ergogenic effects of vitamin D on athletic performance and recovery.* J Int Soc Sports Nutr, 2015. **12**: p. 33.

48. Sale, C., et al., *Carnosine: from exercise performance to health.* Amino Acids, 2013. **44**(6): p. 1477-91.

49. Baye, E., et al., *Physiological and therapeutic effects of carnosine on cardiometabolic risk and disease.* Amino Acids, 2016. **48**(5): p. 1131-49.

50. Boldyrev, A.A., G. Aldini, and W. Derave, *Physiology and pathophysiology of carnosine.* Physiol Rev, 2013. **93**(4): p. 1803-45.

51. Harris, R.C., et al., *The absorption of orally supplied beta-alanine and its effect on muscle carnosine synthesis in human vastus lateralis.* Amino Acids, 2006. **30**(3): p. 279-89.

52. Abe, S., O. Ezaki, and M. Suzuki, *Medium-chain triglycerides (8:0 and 10:0) are promising nutrients for sarcopenia: a randomized controlled trial.* Am J Clin Nutr, 2019. **110**(3): p. 652-665.

53. Abe, S., O. Ezaki, and M. Suzuki, *Medium-Chain Triglycerides in Combination with Leucine and Vitamin D Increase Muscle Strength and Function in Frail Elderly Adults in a Randomized Controlled Trial.* J Nutr, 2016. **146**(5): p. 1017-26.

54. Nishimura, S., et al., *Preventive Effects of the Dietary Intake of Medium-chain Triacylglycerols on Immobilization-induced Muscle Atrophy in Rats.* J Oleo Sci, 2017. **66**(8): p. 917-924.

55. Legault, Z., N. Bagnall, and D.S. Kimmerly, *The Influence of Oral L-Glutamine Supplementation on Muscle Strength Recovery and Soreness Following Unilateral Knee Extension Eccentric Exercise.* Int J Sport Nutr Exerc Metab, 2015. **25**(5): p. 417-26.

56. Amirato, G.R., et al., *L-Glutamine Supplementation Enhances Strength and Power of Knee Muscles and Improves Glycemia Control and Plasma Redox Balance in Exercising Elderly Women.* Nutrients, 2021. **13**(3).

57. Higdon, J. *L-Carnitine.* Micronutrient Information Center. Dietary Factors. 2002 [cited 2021 7/25/2021]; December 2019]. Available from: https://lpi.oregonstate.edu/mic/dietary-factors/L-carnitine.

58. Koozehchian, M.S., et al., *Effects of nine weeks L-Carnitine supplementation on exercise performance, anaerobic power, and exercise-induced oxidative stress in resistance-trained males.* J Exerc Nutrition Biochem, 2018. **22**(4): p. 7-19.

59. Fielding, R., et al., *l-Carnitine Supplementation in Recovery after Exercise.* Nutrients, 2018. **10**(3).

60. Wilkinson, D.J., et al., *Impact of the calcium form of β-hydroxy-β-methylbutyrate upon human skeletal muscle protein metabolism.* Clin Nutr, 2018. **37**(6 Pt A): p. 2068-2075.

61. Stout, J.R., et al., *Effect of calcium β-hydroxy-β-methylbutyrate (CaHMB) with and without resistance training in men and women 65+yrs: a randomized, double-blind pilot trial.* Exp Gerontol, 2013. **48**(11): p. 1303-10.
62. Deutz, N.E., et al., *Effect of β-hydroxy-β-methylbutyrate (HMB) on lean body mass during 10 days of bed rest in older adults.* Clin Nutr, 2013. **32**(5): p. 704-12.
63. Courel-Ibáñez, J., et al., *Effects of β-hydroxy-β-methylbutyrate (HMB) supplementation in addition to multicomponent exercise in adults older than 70 years living in nursing homes, a cluster randomized placebo-controlled trial: the HEAL study protocol.* BMC Geriatrics, 2019. **19**(1): p. 188.
64. Engelen, M.P.K.J. and N.E.P. Deutz, *Is β-hydroxy β-methylbutyrate an effective anabolic agent to improve outcome in older diseased populations?* Current Opinion in Clinical Nutrition & Metabolic Care, 2018. **21**(3): p. 207-213.
65. Jendricke, P., et al., *Specific Collagen Peptides in Combination with Resistance Training Improve Body Composition and Regional Muscle Strength in Premenopausal Women: A Randomized Controlled Trial.* Nutrients, 2019. **11**(4).
66. Zdzieblik, D., et al., *The Influence of Specific Bioactive Collagen Peptides on Body Composition and Muscle Strength in Middle-Aged, Untrained Men: A Randomized Controlled Trial.* Int J Environ Res Public Health, 2021. **18**(9).
67. Zdzieblik, D., et al., *Collagen peptide supplementation in combination with resistance training improves body composition and increases muscle strength in elderly sarcopenic men: a randomised controlled trial.* British Journal of Nutrition, 2015. **114**(8): p. 1237-1245.
68. Oertzen-Hagemann, V., et al., *Effects of 12 Weeks of Hypertrophy Resistance Exercise Training Combined with Collagen Peptide Supplementation on the Skeletal Muscle Proteome in Recreationally Active Men.* Nutrients, 2019. **11**(5).
69. Oikawa, S.Y., et al., *Whey protein but not collagen peptides stimulate acute and longer-term muscle protein synthesis with and without*

resistance exercise in healthy older women: a randomized controlled trial. Am J Clin Nutr, 2020. **111**(3): p. 708-718.

70. Koopman, R., et al., *Glycine metabolism in skeletal muscle: implications for metabolic homeostasis.* Curr Opin Clin Nutr Metab Care, 2017. **20**(4): p. 237-242.

71. Kitakaze, T., et al., *The collagen derived dipeptide hydroxyprolyl-glycine promotes C2C12 myoblast differentiation and myotube hypertrophy.* Biochemical and Biophysical Research Communications, 2016. **478**(3): p. 1292-1297.

Glossary

1RM. The maximun amount of weight that an individual can lift for only one repitition through a full range of motion.

ACCEPTABLE MACRONUTRIENT DISTRIBUTION RANGE (AMDR). The range of intakes of protein, fat, and carbohydrate that is linked to a lower risk of chronic diseases.

ADRENALINE. In the context of muscle health, a hormone released by the adrenal glands to prepare muscles for exercise.

ADVANCED GLYCATION ENDPRODUCTS (AGEs). Damaging compounds that form when proteins or fats bond with sugar in the bloodstream.

AEROBIC METABOLISM. Requires oxygen to generate energy.

ALTERNATE-DAY FASTING (ADF). Alternating calorie-free fasting days with feast days of unlimited consumption of food and beverages.

ALTERNATE-DAY MODIFIED FASTING (ADMF). "Fasting" days consisting of consuming fewer than 25% of daily calorie needs are alternated with feast days of *ad libitum* (liberal) food and beverage consumption.

AMINO ACIDS. The building blocks of protein.

AMP-ACTIVATED PROTEIN KINASE (AMPK). A critical "energy sensor" present in every cell that acts to increase catabolic pathways (breaking down tissues) and decrease anabolic pathways (cell growth and proliferation). Antagonistic to mTOR, it is activated in response to low cellular energy and signals cells to burn excess fat and sugar to recoup energy.

ANABOLIC RESISTANCE. The impaired ability to respond to muscle-building triggers (e.g., amino acids/proteins, insulin, and resistance exercise) that occurs with advancing age.

ANABOLIC. Building up tissue.

ANAEROBIC METABOLISM. Occurs without utilizing oxygen.

ANTIOXIDANT. A compound that protects against oxidative damage to cells caused by unstable, highly reactive free radicals.

ARACHIDONIC ACID (ARA). Whereas this omega-6 fatty acid is a precursor to the synthesis of inflammatory mediators, it is also an important constituent of the membranes of nerve cells that influence neural function.

AUTOPHAGY. A quality-control mechanism whereby damaged proteins and other "expired" cell components are degraded and reutilized for energy or the repair needs of the cell. It literally means "self-eating."

BETA-HYDROXYBUTYRATE (BHB). The predominant ketone in the body.

BRAIN-DERIVED NEUROTROPHIC FACTOR (BDNF). A myokine primarily produced in the brain and also in muscle that is partly responsible for the favorable effect of exercise on cognitive ability as well as depression and anxiety.

BRANCHED-CHAIN AMINO ACIDS (BCAAs). The branched-chain amino acids—leucine, valine, and isoleucine—are three of the nine essential amino acids obtained from the diet; they promote muscle protein synthesis and can also provide energy to muscle cells.

CAFO (CONCENTRATED ANIMAL FEEDING OPERATION). Unlike farming operations that utilize grazing lands, CAFO facilities confine large numbers (thousands) of animals indoors in close proximity with each other.

CARBON CYCLE. A series of cyclical processes in which carbon atoms constantly travel from the atmosphere into organisms in the Earth and then back into the atmosphere.

CARDIORESPIRATORY FITNESS. The ability of the circulatory and respiratory systems to deliver oxygen to muscle mitochondria for energy production during sustained physical activity.

CASSAVA (ALSO CALLED MANIOC AND YUCA; TAPIOCA IS MADE FROM THE SAME ROOT). Native to South America, this starchy root vegetable with a nutty flavor is a major source of carbohydrates in tropical areas of the world.

CATABOLIC. Breaking down tissue.

CATHEPSIN B. A muscle-derived myokine that crosses the blood-brain barrier to induce production of BDNF in the brain and stimulate the formation of new neurons.

COLLAGEN. A structural protein found throughout the body, primarily in connective tissues such as cartilage, bones, tendons, ligaments, and skin.

C-REACTIVE PROTEIN (CRP). A marker of inflammation in the bloodstream.

DOCOSAHEXAENOIC ACID (DHA). An omega-3 fatty acid that plays an essential role in the development of eye and nerve tissue.

EXCESS POST-EXERCISE OXYGEN CONSUMPTION (EPOC). The increased energy expenditure from the afterburn effect that is used to restore the body back to a pre-exercise state and that allows for the aerobic processing (oxidation) of lactate.

EXPENSIVE TISSUE HYPOTHESIS. The increased energy demands of the relatively large human brain are balanced by a corresponding reduction in the size of the equally metabolically expensive (i.e., high-energy-consuming) gut.

FAST-GLYCOLYTIC-OXIDATIVE FIBERS (FOG). A particular subset of fast-twitch muscle fibers that is capable of both anaerobic and aerobic energy production.

FAST-TWITCH MUSCLE FIBERS (TYPE II). A powerful type of muscle fiber especially suited for anaerobic activities such as short, explosive bursts of strength (weightlifting) or speed (sprinting); these fibers fatigue quickly and recover slowly.

FREE RADICALS. Extremely reactive unstable molecules that, when in excess, can cause cellular damage and contribute to many diseases; however, some free radicals are beneficial, e.g., those generated from exercise or from various immune cells.

FUNCTIONAL FOODS. Foods that promote health and help prevent disease in a manner that extends beyond their nutritional impact. Examples include coffee, green tea, olive oil, and beef.

GLUCONEOGENESIS. A process in the body whereby glucose is generated from non-carbohydrate sources such as amino acids, lactate, and glycerol (derived from the breakdown of fats).

GLUT4. A protein that facilitates insulin-stimulated blood glucose transport into muscle and fat cells.

GLUTATHIONE. The body's master antioxidant and detoxifier.

GLYCEMIC INDEX (GI). A measure of how fast a particular food raises blood sugar levels; the GI uses a scale from 1 to 100.

GLYCEMIC LOAD (GL). An estimation of the effect of a carbohydrate food on blood glucose levels based on both the glycemic index and the amount of carbohydrate ingested. The GL is calculated by multiplying the number of available grams of carbohydrate in a serving of a food by the glycemic index and then dividing the total by 100. This is often considered to be a more accurate measurement of a food's impact than its GI number is.

GLYCOGEN. The form of carbohydrates that is stored in the body, primarily in the liver and muscle.

GLYCOLYSIS. The breakdown of sugar to generate energy and pyruvate.

GLYCOLYTIC MUSCLE FIBER. Fibers that use glycolysis to fuel muscle activity (oxygen is not necessary). These are primarily type II muscle fibers.

GREENHOUSE GASES (GHGs). Gases—primarily carbon dioxide, methane, and nitrous oxide—that accumulate in our atmosphere and trap heat from the sun, thus making the planet warmer.

GROWTH HORMONE (GH). A protein made in the pituitary gland that regulates bone growth and collagen synthesis. It is also referred to as human growth hormone (HGH) or somatotropin.

HIGH-INTENSITY INTERVAL TRAINING (HIIT). An effective and time-efficient alternative to traditional aerobic exercise that involves short, intermittent bursts of vigorous exercise interspersed with recovery periods of rest or lower-intensity exercise.

HORMESIS. A process whereby a mild "good" stress—exercising, a short-term lack of food, or getting mild sun exposure—elicits an adaptive beneficial response that increases resilience against more formidable future stressors and promotes resistance to disease.

HYPERCARNIVORE. Animals (including humans) that derive 70% of their food from other animals.

HYPERINSULINEMIA. Elevated levels of insulin in the bloodstream.

HYPERTROPHY (MUSCLE). An increase in muscle size through exercise.

IGF-1 (INSULIN-LIKE GROWTH FACTOR 1). A hormone structurally similar to insulin that is the primary mediator of the growth-promoting effects of growth hormone (GH).

INFLAMMATION (ACUTE). The body's initial healing and repair response to tissue damage or infection. It is characterized by swelling, heat, redness, and pain.

INFLAMMATION (CHRONIC). A response by your immune system that persists beneath the surface after injury or infection and contributes to many chronic diseases.

INITIATION (TRANSLATION). The beginning step in protein synthesis in which mRNA is decoded into proteins.

INSULIN RESISTANCE (IR). The reduced ability of liver, muscle, and fat cells to respond to signals from insulin to take up glucose from the bloodstream.

INTENSITY OF EFFORT. Resistance exercise based on an individual's own effort rather than lifting progressively heavier weights. It involves training with light to moderate weights to the point of muscle failure (fatigue) while maintaining excellent form.

INTERLEUKIN 6 (IL-6). The prototype myokine induced by exercise and linked to many of the benefits of exercise, including the loss of body fat and fat within muscle fibers, anti-inflammatory effects, suppression of tumor growth, appetite inhibition, increased muscle mass and strength in response to resistance training, and improved blood sugar control.

INTERMITTENT FASTING. Taking a break from eating for periods of 12 hours up to potentially several days.

INTERVENTIONAL STUDY. A study designed to evaluate the effect of a specific treatment or preventive measure on outcomes by randomly assigning participants to either the interventional group or a control (placebo) group.

IRISIN. A muscle-derived myokine that crosses the blood-brain barrier to induce production of BDNF in the brain and stimulate the formation of new neurons.

KETOGENESIS. The formation of ketones, primarily in the liver.

KETONE BODY (KETONE). Water-soluble compound produced in the liver as a byproduct of the burning of fat for energy instead of sugar; serves as a major fuel source during fasting/starvation.

KETOSIS. Elevated levels of ketones in the bloodstream.

KREBS CYCLE. A series of reactions occurring in the mitochondria of most living cells in which oxygen is consumed to produce chemical energy (ATP) along with the waste products carbon dioxide and water.

LACTATE. A byproduct of normal metabolism and exercise that is formed when insufficient oxygen is present (anaerobic conditions).

LEGACY EFFECT (METABOLIC MEMORY). In people with diabetes, the long-lasting damage to the body's cells associated with previous periods of high blood sugar.

LEUCINE. The only branched-chain amino acid that *alone* can signal muscle protein synthesis by activating mTOR. The amount of dietary protein needed to trigger mTOR and MPS is dependent on its leucine content.

LIFE-CYCLE ANALYSIS. Determining the environmental impact of a particular service or product (e.g., livestock production, transportation) over the course of its entire life cycle.

LIMITING AMINO ACID. The amino acid present in the lowest amount relative to the amount needed to construct protein. Once a limiting amino acid in a particular protein is used up, muscle protein synthesis comes to a stop.

METABOLIC DISEASE. A disease or disorder that involves abnormal metabolism; that is to say, the abnormal processing or transport of proteins, carbohydrates, or fats.

METABOLIC FLEXIBILITY. A term that describes the ability to periodically transition freely between our two primary fuels—glucose and fat—depending on supply and demand needs.

METABOLIC INFLEXIBILITY. An inability to access and burn fat and ketones for energy—in other words, metabolic *in*flexibility—and the consequent accumulation of body fat.

METABOLIC RESERVE. The body's reserve supply of energy, including protein, that is utilized in times when energy is in high demand (e.g., infection, trauma) or when energy is depleted (e.g., cancer cachexia).

MITOCHONDRIA. Membrane-bound compartments (organelles) within the cell that primarily function to break down food molecules to generate most of the energy needed to power the cell.

MODIFIED KETOGENIC DIET. Unlike the traditional ketogenic diet, this "modified" keto diet puts a premium on dietary protein over ketones.

mTOR (MAMMALIAN TARGET OF RAPAMYCIN). A protein anchoring a powerful signaling pathway that switches on the cellular "machinery" that the body uses to manufacture muscle protein. It signals cells to grow and proliferate.

MUSCLE POWER. The product of strength + speed, this is the ability to exert a force quickly (e.g., when performing explosive jumping, sprinting, or jumping).

MUSCLE PROTEIN SYNTHESIS (MPS). The process that occurs when dietary proteins are broken down via digestion to essential amino acids which are then used to assemble new proteins that are taken up by muscle tissue.

MYOFIBRIL. A long, threadlike strand found in muscle fibers that drives the contraction and relaxation of muscles.

MYOFRIBILLAR PROTEINS. The muscle proteins that comprise the myofibril; these are the primary muscle proteins that respond to resistance exercise by increasing in size.

MYOKINE. Signaling molecules (hormones) produced by muscle cells that exert effects within the muscle itself while also being released into the bloodstream to signal beneficial effects for other organs such as the liver, heart, brain, adipose (fat) tissue, skin, and bone.

MYOSTATIN. An unwanted "reverse" myokine that impairs muscle synthesis and promotes muscle breakdown while also increasing fat mass.

NEOLITHIC PERIOD. The last phase of the Stone Age that started around 10,000 years ago and was marked by the shift from hunting and gathering to agriculture. This period is also known as the Agricultural Revolution.

OBSERVATIONAL (EPIDEMIOLOGICAL) STUDY. A study designed to investigate a research question based solely on observation (as contrasted with an interventional study such as a randomized clinical trial).

OSTEOSARCOPENIA. Coexistence of osteoporosis and sarcopenia.

OXIDATIVE MUSCLE FIBERS. Fibers that rely on a process (aerobic respiration) that requires oxygen to generate energy for muscle contraction. These are primarily type I muscle fibers.

OXIDATIVE STRESS. A harmful condition that develops when the production of free radicals called reactive oxygen species (ROS) exceeds the body's antioxidant defenses.

PALEOLITHIC PERIOD. The earliest period of the Stone Age; extends from approximately 2.5 million years ago to about 10,000 years ago.

***PARANTHROPUS* SPECIES.** A line of human ancestors that continued a dietary trajectory of eating mostly plant foods during the Ice Ages; this species subsequently became extinct.

PERIODIC FASTING (PF). Calorie-free or very-low-calorie fasting periods are cycled for consecutive days ranging from 2 to as many as 21 or more days.

PHYSIOLOGICAL INSULIN RESISTANCE. Our body's way of adapting to a low-carb diet by prioritizing vital glucose for the brain.

PROTEIN DIGESTIBILITY CORRECTED AMINO ACID SCORE (PDCAAS). A method of evaluating the quality of a dietary protein based on human amino acid requirements and the ability of humans to digest the protein.

PSEUDOVITAMIN B12. A compound that is structurally similar to vitamin B12 but is inactive in humans.

PYRUVATE. The end product of the metabolism of glucose via glycolysis; it is transported to the mitochondria to be used in energy production. When oxygen is insufficient, pyruvate is converted to lactate or ethanol.

RANDOMIZED CLINICAL TRIALS (RCTs). Interventional studies that reduce much of the bias linked to observational studies. RCTs are considered to be the gold standard for investigating causal relationships and generating reliable evidence.

REACTIVE OXYGEN SPECIES (ROS). Highly unstable molecules called "free radicals" that are primarily produced in the body as spinoffs of the chemical reactions in the cellular mitochondria that convert food and oxygen to energy.

RESISTANCE TRAINING (RT). A conditioning strategy that involves working against some type of external resistance (load) in a progressive manner.

RESTING METABOLIC RATE. The rate at which the body burns energy (calories) when at complete rest.

RUMINANTS. Animals with two-toed feet that chew their cud and have four-chambered stomachs, e.g., cattle, sheep.

SARCOPENIA. Age-related loss of muscle mass and muscle strength.

SATELLITE CELLS. Precursors to muscle cells (or muscle fibers); also known as muscle stem cells.

SATURATED FATTY ACIDS. Fats that are typically solid at room temperature, e.g., butterfat, beef fat, and lard.

SIRTUINS. A family of enzymes that has been shown to extend lifespan in yeast and mice. Sirtuins mediate the health benefits of exercise, including reduced oxidative stress and inflammation, creation of new muscle mitochondria and enhanced mitochondrial function, and improved DNA repair capability.

SLOW-TWITCH MUSCLE FIBERS (TYPE I). Muscle fibers ideally suited for low-intensity endurance (aerobic) exercise since they're packed with blood vessels, mitochondria, and oxygen-binding myoglobin; these fibers are slow to fatigue and recover quickly.

SPRINT INTERVAL TRAINING (SIT). A more demanding version of HIIT that involves repeated 30-second "all-out" (supramaximal) efforts followed by longer recovery periods of 4 – 5 minutes.

TIME-RESTRICTED FEEDING (TRF). Eating within narrow time windows (typically 4 – 12 hours) while fasting for periods of 12 – 20 hours.

TUMOR NECROSIS FACTOR ALPHA (TNF-α). A marker of inflammation in the bloodstream.

UNSATURATED FATTY ACIDS. Fats that are usually liquid at room temperature, i.e., oils.

VO2 MAX. The maximum capacity of the body to transport (via circulation) and utilize oxygen during intense or maximal exercise.

Index

About the Author

Robert Iafelice, MS, RDN is a functional nutritionist and free-lance medical writer. He has contributed several chapters to the 6th edition of Disease Prevention and Treatment, a medical reference book of evidence-based protocols used to combat the diseases of aging. He has also written continuing education programs for nutrition professionals, including Intermittent Fasting: Evidence-Based Approaches to Optimized Health and Disease Resistance and Clinical Strategies to Combat Food Allergies and Intolerances.

Robert received a Bachelor of Arts degree in Chemistry from Miami University in Oxford, Ohio, and a Master of Science degree in Nutrition Science from Case Western Reserve University in Cleveland, Ohio. Most of his experience as a practicing registered dietitian was in the field of integrative/functional medicine with a focus on food allergy.

Robert's diverse background also includes extensive experience in fitness/wellness as a gym owner, university nutrition instructor, and health educator in the nutraceuticals industry. He also has experience in the field of oncology. As a fitness enthusiast, he competes in Masters Track & Field events.

For more information, visit: hold-on-to-your-muscle.com.